Department of
Homeland Security
**United States
Coast Guard**

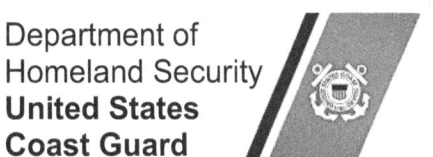

Coast Guard Medical Manual
Volume II

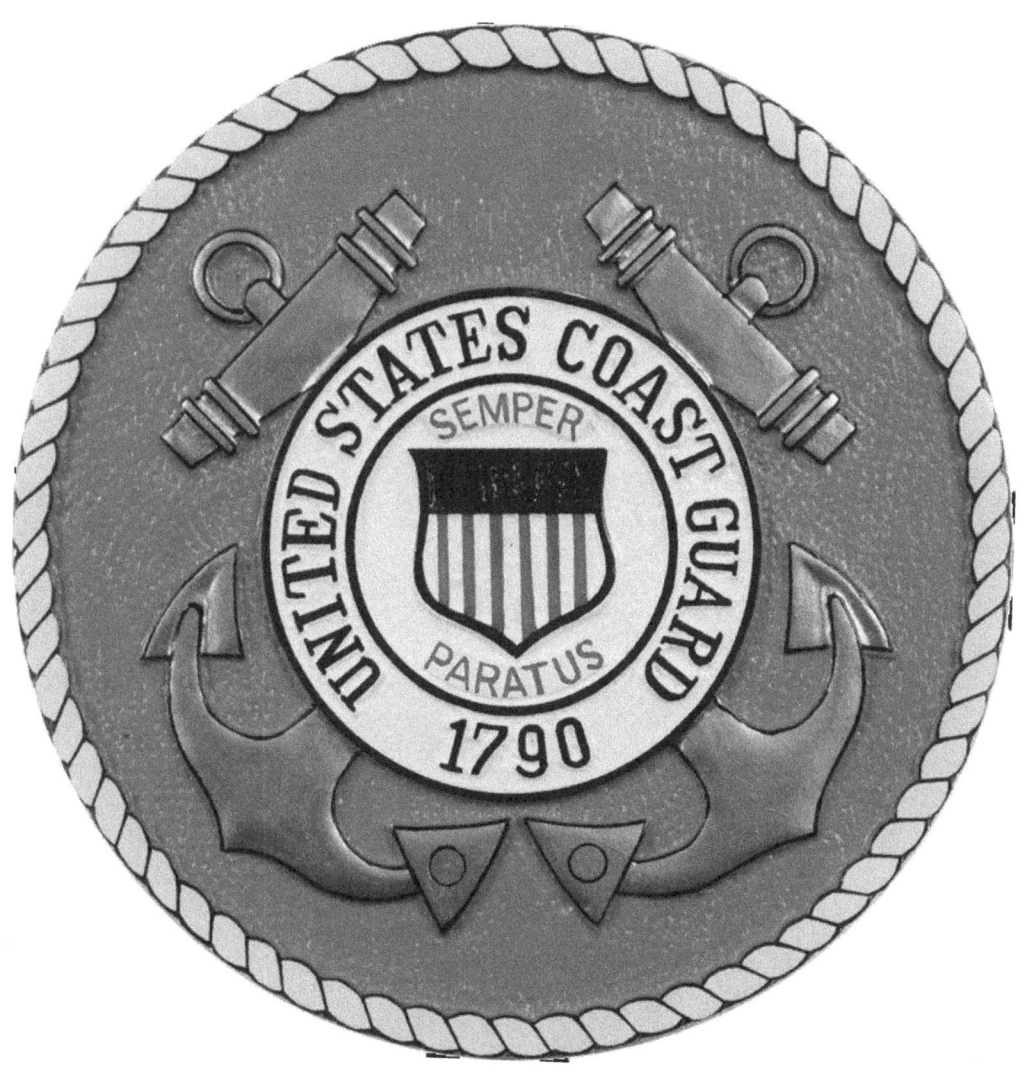

**COMDINST M6000.1F
JUNE 2018**

Medical Manual

Table of Contents

Volume 2

CHAPTER 8

FISCAL AND SUPPLY MANAGEMENT

CHAPTER 9

HEALTH SERVICES TECHNICIANS ASSIGNED TO INDEPENDENT DUTY

Section A. Independent Duty Afloat.

Section B. Independent Duty Ashore at Sectors, Sector Field Offices, Air Stations, and Small Boat Stations.

CHAPTER 10
PHARMACY OPERATIONS AND DRUG CONTROL

Section A. Pharmacy Administration.

Section B. Controlled Substances.

Section C. Forms and Records.

Section D. Drug Dispensing Without a Medical Officer.

CHAPTER 11
HEALTH CARE PROCUREMENT

Section A. Contracting For Health Care Services.

Section B. Health Care Services Invoice Review and Auditing.

Section C. Claims Processing.

CHAPTER 12

OCCUPATIONAL MEDICAL SURVEILLANCE AND EVALUATION PROGRAM (OMSEP)

Section A. **Information on OMSEP.**

CHAPTER 13

QUALITY IMPROVEMENT

Section M. Patient Affairs Program.

CHAPTER 14

MEDICAL INFORMATION SYSTEM (MIS) PROGRAM

Section A. Medical Information Systems (MIS) Plan.

Section B. Medical Information System.

Section C. Medical Readiness Reporting System (MRRS).

Section D. Medical Information Implementation Guide (MIIG)

CHAPTER 8

FISCAL AND SUPPLY MANAGEMENT

CHAPTER EIGHT – FISCAL AND SUPPLY MANAGEMENT

A. <u>Resource Management</u>.

1. <u>CG Headquarters</u>.

   a. Commandant (CG-11) obtains health services program resources from the budget process for these purposes:

      (1) Ensures AFC-57 funds are expended in accordance with the Financial Resource Management Manual, COMDTINST M7100.3 (series).

      (2) Targeting AFC-57 and AFC-73 funds to pay the Department of Defense for all health care the Army, Navy, Air Force, TRICARE and USMTF programs provided to CG beneficiaries.

      (3) Targeting AFC-57 funds to HSWL to pay for all non-Federal and VA medical care provided in each region.

      (4) All purchases of medical equipment or devises which connect to the Commandant (CG-1) data network must be approved by Commandant (CG-1123).

      (5) Targeting AFC-57 funds to HSWL SC to acquire health care equipment.

      (6) Targeting AFC-57 funds to allotted units in response to budget requests to HSWL SC.

   b. <u>In charge of health care facilities</u>. Commandant (CG-11) is also the Program Manager for replacing, expanding, or creating health care facilities with Acquisition, Construction, and Improvement Appropriation funds and works with Commandant (CG-924) and the Lant Area Facilities Design and Construction Center staffs on plans and layouts.

2. <u>Health, Safety, and Work-Life Service Center (HSWL SC)</u>. HSWL SC administers the health services program in their respective area of responsibility. Administrative functions include:

   a. Approving and funding care provided by non-Federal and Department of Veterans Affairs sources.

   b. <u>Health care equipment</u>. Approving or disapproving requests to procure health care equipment costing more than $5,000.00 for units with CG Clinics/AFC-57 funding and over $3,500.00 for sickbays with HS's assigned via AFC-57 funding; (See Paragraph 8.D)

c. Approving clinic budgets. Each clinic shall submit a zero-based AFC-57 direct care funding request to HSWL SC through their RM. This request should include predicted equipment procurement requests to Commandant (CG-83) using the automated ATU budget process according to current directives. The HSWL SC request should include a line item for each clinic, proposed equipment funding, and an estimate of non-Federal health care costs.

3. Regional Manager's (RM) Responsibility.

a. RM's Responsibility. A Regional Manager (RM) is charged with ensuring that all aspects of his/her health care facilities operate effectively and efficiently. This means using personnel, funds, equipment, expendable supplies and materials, health care spaces, and external health care providers economically and efficiently. The RM oversees all health care equipment maintenance. Regional Managers will ensure that management of command resources provides the best amount of care to all eligible beneficiaries at the least possible cost to the Government.

b. Reports. The unit Regional Manager directly controls the unit's financial plan or budget, including unit health care resources. By the 5th working day of each month, the Regional Manager reports medical, dental, pharmaceutical and equipment operating targets, adjustments to the targets, and actual expenditures to HSWL SC for inclusion in the monthly report forwarded to Commandant (CG-112). From an oversight or management review perspective, repeated or recurring amounts of unit Fund Code-57 (AFC-57) monies dedicated to health care are the "base" funds. Regional Managers must justify additional unit operating funds above this base solely on the criterion of increased workloads or mission support.

c. Review of funds. The Regional Manager will review all uses of unit funds and reallocate funds during the current fiscal year. The Regional Manager must first inform the chain of command before he/she can reduce the amount of care the unit's clinic provides to eligible beneficiaries. The RM will report the circumstances supporting the decision and identify what resources are required to ensure normal health care facility operations through the end of the fiscal year. The HSWL SC will address these current fiscal year AFC-57 facilities requests.

B. General Property Management and Accountability.

   1. Basic Policies. The Director of Health, Safety and Work-Life shall:

      a. Manage accounts. Establish procedures to manage and account for health care material pursuant to the personal property management policies contained in the U. S. Coast Guard Property Management Manual, COMDTINST M4500.5 (series).

      b. Direct and coordinate the health care supply system;

      c. Determine requirements for health care material; and,

      d. Establish allowance lists, advise, and assist field units.

   2. Physical Property Classifications. Property is divided into two categories: real property and personal property. Health care material is personal property and is accounted for in accordance with U. S. Coast Guard Property Management Manual, COMDTINST M4500.5 (series).

   3. Property Responsibility and Accountability.

      a. Health Services Administrators. Health Services Administrators are responsible for the accountability of the property for their facilities. Additionally, they serve as the health services finance and supply officer.

      b. In the absence of a Health Services Administrators, the senior commissioned health services department representative acts as the property custodian.

      c. If Health Services Technicians only are assigned to a facility, the senior Health Services Technician acts as the property custodian.

   4. Expending Property Unnecessarily. All persons having custody of health care property shall avoid any unnecessary expenditures of such property within their authority's limits and shall prevent such expenditures by others.

   5. Stock Levels, Reorder Points, and Stock Limits.

      a. General. Stock levels, reorder points, and stock limits discussed below apply to all health care facilities, especially those at major shore units (i.e. HQs units) such as the Academy, TRACEN Petaluma, TRACEN Yorktown, and Training Center Cape May. These large facilities with multiple components (e.g., pharmacy, laboratory, dental clinic, etc.) need to maintain a greater stock depth to serve their beneficiaries. U. S. Coast Guard Property Management Manual, COMDTINST M4500.5 (series) contains overall supply policy and procedures.

b. Terms.

    (1) Operating Stock. That quantity of material on hand needed to meet daily operating needs during the interval between delivery of replenishments.

    (2) Safety Stock. That amount of inventory in addition to operating stock needed to sustain operations if deliveries are delayed or demands unexpectedly heavy.

    (3) Reorder Point (Low Limit). Both terms mean the predetermined inventory level for a specific item at which it is reordered.

c. Stock Inventory and Transactions. All health care facilities shall maintain sufficient amounts of stock to prevent out-of-stock conditions. To do so, maintain stock inventory and transaction records, either electronically or by using stock cards, inventory records, etc.

    (1) Generally, health services supply activities at facilities with multiple components are authorized one month's safety stock. Experience may prove this level is not adequate for certain items or in certain circumstances. These units are authorized to maintain a larger supply if and wherever exceptional circumstances dictate. Establish procedures to ensure review of stock records periodically to identify items reaching a low limit (reorder point), the authorized allowance, and quantity to revise low limits if current usage so indicates.

    (2) Ships and small shore units may use the minimum quantities indicated in the Health Services Allowance List to establish reorder points. If the list does not indicate a minimum allowance, e.g. for "optional" items, establish reorder points for commonly used items based on current usage rates. Do not order excessive quantities of material.

    (3) When a ship receives orders to deploy or a station notice of a change in operating conditions that may require additional material, promptly review authorized allowance quantities to replenish critical items in time for the deployment or operational change.

    (4) Pharmacies procuring drugs through prime vendor systems (either directly or through pharmacy officer staffed clinics) should try to stock one-month quantities of regularly used items. Ongoing inventories of these limited quantities are not required except where applicable for controlled substances. Pharmacies shall "sight inventory" monthly before ordering.

6. Transferring and Loaning Property. Written approval is required from Commandant (CG-112) to loan health care property to any state, community, organization, or private individual. Property transferred to other military units is at the Regional Manager's discretion. Obtain custody receipts in such

instances. A Requisition and Invoice/Shipping Document, Form DD-1149 shall be used to transfer property locally, and from one activity to another according to the U. S. Coast Guard Property Management Manual, COMDTINST M4500.5 (series)

C. Custody, Issues, and Disposition.

1. Transferring Custody. When transferring custody of health services property and supplies a joint inventory is required conducted by both the departing and relieving custodians and an independent person who has no direct interest in the inventory outcome. If a joint inventory is impossible, the departing custodian shall conduct an inventory and submit a written report to the Regional Manager before departing. As soon as possible after reporting, the relieving custodian also shall conduct an inventory, report the same to the Regional Manager, and indicate any discrepancies noted between the two. In both cases, the inventories should include the participation of an independent person. Additionally, in all cases, an acknowledgment of inventory correctness must be entered in the unit Health Services Log. (See "Pharmacy Operations and Drug Control," Chapter 10 of this Manual, for detailed information on controlled substances).

2. Storerooms.

   a. Bulk stock. At large facilities, bulk stock of health care supplies and materials used by the various facility components (e.g., pharmacy, laboratory, dental clinic, etc.) shall be kept in a specifically designated storeroom. If facility layout permits, it may be advantageous to permit designated individuals responsible for a particular component (pharmacy, dental clinic, etc.) to manage their area's expendable supplies. The individual responsible for medical supply shall process their procurement requests. Otherwise, manage clinic supplies from a designated storeroom.

   b. Supply person. An individual familiar with supply procedures shall be in charge of the storeroom. He/she shall report directly to a Health Services Administrator.

   c. Procurement request. In the interest of proper management, centralize clinic procurement request processing. Health Services Administrator shall verify all procurement requests, including prime vendor "ZOA" documents, to ensure funds are available in their respective clinic's budget allocation.

3. Issuing Material.

   a. Supplies issued by or removed from the storeroom should be immediately recorded on the appropriate stock record. In large facilities where the health services storeroom is a distinct organizational entity, stores issued shall be made only upon receiving a properly prepared and authenticated local requisition document.

   b. Use the Requisition and Invoice/Shipping Document, Form DD-1149 to issue, return, or transfer equipment between activity components.

4. Inspecting Storerooms.

   a. Health services store items require periodic inspection (every three months for consumable supplies and equipment) to detect signs of deterioration or expiration. Accomplish such inspections by physically examining representative samples of various age groups of stock on hand.

b. It is extremely important to issue oldest stock first ("First in, First out"). This is true of all items but is mandatory for potency-dated items and those subject to spoilage.

5. <u>Disposing of Property</u>.

a. In disposing of health services personal property, follow the U. S. Coast Guard Property Management Manual, COMDTINST M4500.5 (series) procedures regardless of the circumstances or conditions requiring disposal (e.g., over-ordering, decline in demand, fair wear and tear requiring survey, or damage requiring replacement).

b. Certain conditions may require Board of Survey action. U. S. Coast Guard Property Management Manual, COMDTINST M4500.5 (series) contains procedures for this action.

c. Expired or contaminated drugs should be disposed of in accordance with Chapter 10 of this manual.

d. Do not dispose of medical materials at sea. Prepare materials for disposal and retain them onboard in a secure area until disposed of in accordance with Federal, State, and local laws.

e. Commandant Notices and other directives requiring disposal of defective material constitute authorization to immediately dispose of any suspect items on hand.

D. Health Services Supply System.

1. Health Services Control Point. Commandant (CG-112) is the Health Services Control Point for CG health care material; in that capacity they:

   a. Prepare and distribute the Health Services Allowance List, Ashore, COMDTINST M6700.5 (series), Health Services Allowance List, Afloat, COMDTINST M6700.6 (series), and Health Services Allowance List, Shore Units and Vessels, COMDTINST M6700.7 (series).

   b. Inform and assist field units.

   c. Review and respond to requests to change units' base operating funds allotment targets. Annually provides funds for routine health care supplies to the field as part of the recurring base of funds distributed through the Administrative Target Unit (ATU) budget process.

2. Responsibility for General Stores Items.

   a. Supply Officer.

      (1) Procures, receives, stores, issues, ships, transfers, and accounts for command stores and equipment;

      (2) Maintains specified records; and,

      (3) Submits required reports for stores and equipment.

   b. Health Services Department Representative. Except where specific responsibility has been assigned, the Health Services Department Representative does not determine general supply requirements but acts in an advisory capacity for those items the department uses. The Health Services Department Representative will maintain close contact with the Supply Officer on special department needs and advise the latter when the requirement for any item will exceed the quantity normally carried in stock. The individual designated in writing as responsible for Health Services supply operations shall maintain a supply policy and procedures manual.

3. Supply Support Assistance.

   a. Direct problems with supply support of health care supplies that cannot be resolved through the supply source, to HSWL SC.

   b. Commandant (CG-1123) will coordinate initial outfitting of new classes of units and vessels, billeted with an HS, with pharmaceuticals when requested by the project manager through Commandant (CG-DCMS-831). The project manager will provide an AC&I line of accounting to the HSWL SC. The HSWL SC will direct a clinic to purchase and hold the pharmaceuticals until the cutter's HS reports aboard and can take appropriate custody.

4. <u>Authorized Allowances</u>. CG units are assigned specific minimum required allowances of health care supplies and equipment as described in the Health Services Allowance List, Ashore, COMDTINST M6700.5 (series), Health Services Allowance List, Afloat, COMDTINST M6700.6 (series), and Health Services Allowance List, Shore Units and Vessels, COMDTINST M6700.7 (series).

5. <u>Supply Sources</u>.

   a. <u>Standard Items</u>. Items listed in the DoD Medical Catalog (FEDLOG) are "standard". Obtain items with an Advice Acquisition Code (AAC) of "D" from the Defense Personnel Support Center (DPSC) through the Automated Requisition Management System (ARMS).

   (1) Non-Obtain "non-standard" items, i.e., those not described as above, from commercial sources.

   (2) All commercial procurements shall be made under the applicable acquisition regulations and Coast Guard Acquisition Procedures (CGAP), COMDTINST M4200.19 (series). Commercial procurement of health care supplies, equipment, and repair and maintenance service is authorized in these conditions:

      (a) Time does not permit obtaining standard items from Government sources; or,

      (b) A legitimate need exists for nonstandard items;

      (c) Equipment requires repair or maintenance.

   (3) These items are authorized:

      (a) Newly listed standard items not available from government sources;

      (b) Necessary non-standard health care supplies and equipment;

      (c) Medical Catalog (FEDLOG) items bearing the Acquisition Advice Code "L";

      (d) Equipment repair and maintenance (excluding installation); and

      (e) Health care technical books, publications, and professional journals.

   (4) Local or commercial procurement is not authorized for these items:

      (a) Non-standard items differing only slightly from standard items of identical capability; and

(b) Preferred trade names and proprietary products in lieu of standard items.

b. Prime Vendor Items.

(1) A prime vendor is one pre-arranged on behalf of the government procurement system. The Defense Personnel Support Center (DPSC) negotiates prime vendors, equivalent to Federal "depot" sources, for medical commodities.

(2) Where available, DPSC prime vendors shall serve as the primary source of supply for pharmaceuticals. Use other sources if it is determined their price or service better meet the unit's needs.

6. Health Care Equipment.

a. Factors for Initial Procurement. Due to changes in the beneficiary population or unit mission, a health care facility may require health care equipment not previously held by that facility. Units requesting an initial procurement shall provide justification on a U.S. Coast Guard Health Care Equipment Request, Form CG-5211.

b. New Installations. The appropriate construction project (AC&I) funds normally will pay for equipment for newly constructed facilities. To ensure standardization, authorization and approval MUST be obtained from Commandant (CG-112) before requisitioning or procuring health care equipment for new installations.

c. Health Care Equipment. All units with health care equipment (items with an original cost of more than $5,000.00 or more for clinics and $3,500.00 or more for sickbays) shall verify their equipment annually (January) and submit the report to HSWL SC. Definitions for health care equipment, procurement procedures, and the criteria used for approval are outlined below.

(1) Health care equipment. Any item of health care equipment which meets the following criteria:

(a) Costs $5,000.00 or more for clinics and $3,500.00 or more for sickbays.

(b) Does not lose its identity when installed or placed into service.

(c) Has a life expectancy of one year or more.

(2) Units shall submit requests for health care equipment on a U.S. Coast Guard Health Care Equipment Request, Form CG-5211 to HSWL SC. If the HSWL SC is unable to evaluate the U.S. Coast Guard Health Care Equipment Request, Form CG-5211 within 15 working days of receipt,

HSWL SC shall notify the requesting unit regarding the delay. HSWL SC shall review the request and provide a forwarding endorsement that, as a minimum, addresses the following areas:

(a) How the equipment is or is not appropriate for the requesting health care facility.

(b) Why the purchase is or is not cost effective.

(c) How the equipment will or will not impact on the quality of patient care.

(3) HSWL SC will evaluate health care equipment requests, and within 30 days of receipt of the U.S. Coast Guard Health Care Equipment Request, Form CG-5211 will notify the unit that one of the following actions will be taken:

(a) Purchase of the requested equipment.

(b) Purchase of a substitute item of a different make or model in order to standardize health care equipment and/or ensure cost effectiveness.

(c) Return the request via the chain of command with an explanation of why the equipment request was disapproved.

(4) Health care equipment costing less than $5,000.00 for clinics and less than $3,500.00 for sickbays is a unit responsibility and shall be purchased using unit AFC-57 funds.

7. Emergency Procurement. A request for an emergency procurement may be relayed to the HSWL SC by telephone, followed by a faxed copy of a completed form U.S. Coast Guard Health Care Equipment Request, Form CG-5211.

8. Factors for Replacing Equipment. The fact that an item of health care equipment is approaching, or has passed, its normal life expectancy is not considered sufficient cause for replacement in and of itself. Units that request replacement equipment shall provide justification on the U.S. Coast Guard Health Care Equipment Request, Form CG-5211. Factors which are considered sufficient cause for equipment replacement include any of the following:

a. Unreliability. Documented unreliability of equipment, demonstrated by unusual maintenance expenses or high frequency of repairs.

b. Excessive repair costs, onetime or repetitive.

c. Obsolete Equipment. Equipment is obsolete and new technology exists that reduces pain and discomfort, improves treatment, increases diagnostic accuracy, significantly reduces costs by conserving personnel, supplies, or utilities, or increases efficiency by reducing patient treatment time.

d. Receipts.

(1) The unit shall retain one copy of signed receipts for health services material for record purposes.

(2) Send one copy of signed receipts for all health care equipment to HSWL SC.

(3) Maintain copies of receipts for controlled substances and security materials separately for record purposes.

e. Maintenance.

(1) Each unit is responsible for maintaining health care equipment in optimum, safe operating condition. Maintenance shall include:

(a) Measures necessary to ensure the equipment's operating safety and efficiency (preventive maintenance);

(b) Manufacturer's representatives' required checks to meet warranty requirements;

(c) Removing from service if deficiencies are detected; and

(d) Replacing defective parts.

(2) Preventive maintenance is systematic inspection of and service to equipment to maintain it in optimum operating condition. A properly executed program will detect and correct minor problems before they render the equipment inoperable. Manufacturers usually require preventive maintenance to maintain the warranty. Maintenance records are also valuable tools for evaluating equipment needs and justifying future equipment procurement requests.

(3) Each clinic shall designate a Preventive Maintenance Coordinator who ensures the program is established and functions effectively. If a Biomedical Equipment Repair Technician (BMET) is assigned to the unit, he/she fills this role. Clinics may contract for preventive maintenance services if funding permits and are encouraged to enter into cooperative agreements with DoD MTFs whenever possible. Each unit shall:

(a) Establish a preventive maintenance schedule for all health care equipment. Each unit shall determine maintenance intervals based on manufacturers' recommendations and frequency of use.

(b) Maintain a written record of all preventive maintenance and repairs performed on health care equipment using a Medical/Dental Equipment Maintenance Record, Form NAVMED 6700-3CG. Use side A to record preventive maintenance and safety checks and side B to record repairs.

(c) Charge health care equipment maintenance costs to unit AFC-57 funds.

(d) HSWL SC and HQ units shall establish and maintain a program to replace their health care equipment.

E. Eyeglasses and Ophthalmic Services.

    1. General. This section describes ophthalmic services (refractions and spectacle issue) provided.

    2. Personnel Authorized Refractions.

        a. CG health care facilities and USMTFs. CG health care facilities and USMTFs to the extent of available facilities, including ophthalmologists' and optometrists' services, may furnish refractions to active duty and dependents not enrolled in TRICARE Prime on a "space available" basis and retired uniformed services members.

        b. No MTF. When USMTF's are not available, HSWL SC may authorize refractions at other facilities for active duty members only.

        c. USMTFs may furnish non-active duty eligible beneficiaries refractions if facilities are available. USMTFs may not furnish eyeglasses to dependents at government expense except as Section 8.E.3.b.(2)(b) authorizes.

        d. Reserve members on active duty for training for more than 30 days are authorized repair or replacement of standard eyeglasses during the active duty period.

    3. Procuring and Issuing Standard Prescription Eyewear.

        a. CG units shall order standard eyewear from optical laboratories as outlined in this section.

            (1) Civilian sources are acceptable for procuring eyewear providing the prescription is for standard frames and lenses are available from fabrication labs. Transcribe this request onto a Eyewear Prescription, Form DD-771.

            (2) If fabrication would entail a prolonged delay (more than eight weeks) and the member's vision is so poor he/she cannot safely perform assigned duties, procure non-standard eyewear from local civilian sources using non-Federal health care funds.

            (3) Members requiring corrective lenses shall have two pair at all times, including eyeglasses issued from government sources or purchased at their own expense.

            (4) Requests for tinted eyewear for non-aviation members must be justified solely on the duties they perform, e.g. majority of duty time in bright sunlight, etc.

            (5) Replacement eyewear may be obtained without repeating a visual acuity check, provided the replacement prescription is less than two years old. If a corrected visual acuity check is required and indicates the current prescription is inadequate, patient must obtain a refraction.

        b. Available Eyewear and Standard Eyewear Sources of Supply.

            (1) These types of eyewear are available:

Type of Correction	Cellulose acetate frame	
	Glass Lens	Plastic Lens
Single Vision, white [1]	X	X
Single Vision, tinted [1,2]	X	X
Bifocal, 25mm segment, white [1]	X	X
Bifocal, 25mm segment, tinted [1,2]	X	X
Trifocal, white	X	
Cataract Aspheric		X
Trifocal, white and tinted [1,2]		X
(1) Eyewear provided in FG-58 (Flight Goggle) mounting for authorized personnel (2) Only N-15 and N-32 tints authorized		

Table 8-E-1

(2) Process all requests for standard prescription eyewear through the below military optical laboratory. This is the only optical laboratory from which CG units are authorized to order standard prescription eyewear.

Naval Ophthalmic Support and Training Activity Yorktown, VA 23691-5071

Table 8-E-2

(a) It is extremely important to properly complete the Eyewear Prescription, Form DD-771 service identification block to indicate the patient's service affiliation.

(b) Dependent care in isolated areas. Spectacles may be furnished to command-sponsored dependents of uniformed services members assigned outside CONUS with the exception of Alaska, Hawaii and Puerto Rico.

(3) Procurement Procedures. Order all prescription eyewear using the Eyewear Prescription, Form DD-771. It is extremely important to accurately complete the prescription form. If the prescription is wrong the patient is inconvenienced. The CG is required to pay for eyewear even if it cannot be used. The supply activity will reject an improperly prepared prescription, resulting in delay. Use these guidelines to prepare a Eyewear Prescription, Form DD-771. See Section 4-B for more detailed instructions.

(a) Use a separate Eyewear Prescription, Form DD-771 for each type of eyewear.

(b) If no health services personnel are available at the unit, send the prescription obtained from the health record or local civilian source to the health record custodian to prepare and submit the Eyewear Prescription, Form DD-771.

(c) Submit all three Eyewear Prescription, Form DD-771 copies to the approving authority or supply activity; disregard the distribution instructions. Remove all carbon sheets before submission. File a photocopy of the Eyewear Prescription, Form DD-771 in the member's health record.

(d) TRACEN Cape May shall send recruits' eyewear prescriptions separately and mark the envelope, "RECRUIT—PLEASE EXPEDITE".

(4) Health Record Entries. Record on a separate Eyewear Prescription, Form DD-771 the current prescription, including frame measurements and all other data necessary to reorder eyewear, for each individual requiring eyeglasses.

4. Aviation Prescription Lenses. Aviation personnel are authorized two pair of clear aviation spectacles (FG-58) and one pair of tinted spectacles (N-15).

   a. Aviators Engaged in Actual Flight Operations. Aviation spectacles may be ordered for distant vision correction, or for distant vision and near vision correction (bifocal lenses). Those aviation personnel engaged in flight operation who desire near vision only correction in aviation frames must order bifocal lenses containing plano top portion and the near vision correction on the bottom. Spectacles containing only near vision correction are not authorized in aviation frames. This type correction will only be order in cellulose acetate frames.

   b. Landing Signal Officers (LSO).

   c. CG Ceremonial Honor Guard personnel.

   d. Small Boat Crew members are required to wear a helmet while performing their assigned duties.

5. Contact Lenses. Contact lenses are issued only to active duty personnel for postocular surgical difficulties or to enable a member to overcome a handicapping disease or impairment. HSWL SC will not approve contact lenses solely for cosmetic reasons with exception of the CG Honor Guard, where wearing of eye glasses may interfere with the performance of their duties.

   a. Submit letter requests for contact lenses to HSWL SC under Section 2-A-7.a.; include the type of lenses and cost.

   b. Approval. If HSWL SC approves they will provide an authorization number by return correspondence. Units will write this number on all correspondence and billings before submitting to HSWL SC.

6. <u>Sunglasses for Polar Operations</u>. Military fabrication laboratories no longer issue polar operation sunglasses. Activities requiring such glasses may use the process below to obtain them:

    a. <u>Non-prescription Lenses</u>. If issuing, the command must purchase and issue non-prescription lenses as part of the cold weather clothing allowance and pay the lenses' costs from operating expenses. The command should issue the lenses on a custodial basis, departing members should return them to the command for reissue.

    b. <u>Prescription Lenses</u>. Procure prescription lenses from NOSTRA.

        (1) Aviation-type frames.

        (2) Lenses must contain Type 1 or 1-A metallic coat.

7. <u>Safety Glasses</u>.

    a. <u>Standards</u>. Non-prescription or prescription safety glasses meeting American National Standards Institute Standard Z87.1 shall be for industrial wear to military and civilian personnel working in any environment hazardous to eyes, e.g., welders, machinists, mechanics, riggers, and grinders.

    b. Non-prescription safety glasses shall be furnished on a custody receipt when a prescription lenses are not required.

    c. Prescription safety glasses are no longer available from military optical laboratories. Prescription safety glasses are only issued to personnel with a current eye exam within the last 12 months and costs incurred are chargeable to unit funds.

        (1) Military personnel prescription safety eyewear will be purchased utilizing AFC-57 funds.

        (2) Civilian personnel prescription safety eyewear will not be purchased utilizing AFC-57 funds.

CHAPTER 9

HEALTH SERVICES TECHNICIANS ASSIGNED TO INDEPENDENT DUTY

Section A. Independent Duty Afloat.

Section B. Independent Duty Ashore at Sectors, Sector Field Offices, Air Stations, and Small Boat Stations.

Section C. Independent Duty in Support of Deployable Specialized Forces

Section D. Quality Improvement Compliance Program (QICP)

Section E. Independent Duty Management of TRICARE

CHAPTER NINE – HEALTH SERVICES TECHNICIANS ASSIGNED TO INDEPENDENT DUTY

Section A. Independent Duty Afloat.

1. Introduction. An Independent Duty Health Services Technician (IDHS) is a Health Services Technician (HS) assigned to a unit that has no attached Medical Officer (MO). An Independent Duty Health Services (IDHS) Afloat is a Health Services Technician assigned to a cutter. The identification or term Independent Duty Health Services Technician, used in any form, only identifies those Health Services Technicians that have successfully completed one of the three recognized Independent Duty Training courses, i.e. the USCG Independent Duty Health Services Technician, USN Independent Duty Corpsman, or USAF Independent Duty Medical Technician courses. Assignment to independent duty is challenging. The role is one of tremendous responsibility.

2. Mission, General Duties and Responsibilities.

   a. Mission. The Health Services Technician serving independently is charged with the responsibility for the prevention and control of disease and injury, and the treatment of the sick and injured.

   b. General Duties. HSs on independent duty perform the administrative duties and, to the extent for which qualified, the clinical duties prescribed for MOs of vessels. (See United States Coast Guard Regulations 1992, COMDTINST M5000.3 (series) and Section 1-B of this Manual.). They shall not attempt, nor be required to provide, health care for which they are not trained and qualified. They shall provide care only for AD personnel; however they may provide care to non-active duty patients on an emergency basis. The filling of prescriptions for other than AD personnel shall be strictly limited to emergency situations and to authorized stock on hand under the allowance list for the unit. They may, under the guidance set in Chapter 10 of this Manual, establish non-prescription medication programs for eligible beneficiaries.

   c. Responsibilities. The Commanding Officer (CO) is responsible for the health and readiness of the command. The health services department is charged with advising the CO of conditions existing that may be detrimental to the health of personnel and for making appropriate recommendations for correcting such conditions. Meticulous attention to all details and aspects of preventing disease must be a continuing program. It is imperative that shipboard sanitation and preventive health practices be reviewed constantly in order that any disease promoting situation may be discovered immediately and promptly eradicated. In the absence of a permanently attached MO the vessel's Executive Officer (XO) will have direct administrative responsibility for medical matters when no MO is attached to the vessel. The role of the IDHS is to assist the command in maintaining the good health and physical readiness of the crew. To accomplish this, the IDHS must be informed of planned operations and anticipate any operational demands resulting from such operations. To this end, the IDHS will consult and advise the command in all matters with potential to effect crew readiness or the health of personnel. Some of the duties of the IDHS include but are not limited to:

(1) IDHSs are recognized as a critical component to managing the CG wellness home for active duty members empanelled both indirectly and directly to practice sites. In essence, the IDHS facilitates the "wellness home away from home" and serves as the conduit to the Regional Practice.

(2) Assessment and treatment of illness and injury. Hold daily sick call. Diagnose and treat patients within capabilities. Fully document care in the electronic health record and request cosignature of 100 percent of records by the DMOA. When indicated, refer cases to facilities where Medical or Dental Officers are available or, if this is not practical, obtain help and advice by radio or other expeditious means.

(3) Prevention of illness and injury through an aggressive environmental health program. Such a program includes inspection of living and working spaces, food service and storage areas, handling practices, integrated pest management practices, potable water quality surveillance, and recognition and management of communicable diseases.

(4) Provision of Health Services training aligned with the needs and mission of the unit.

(5) Security and proper use of health services supplies, material and property.

(6) Maintenance and documentation of medical and dental readiness of unit personnel. The IDHS will assist the command in ensuring the medical and dental readiness for the personnel in their AOR by providing monthly Medical and Dental Readiness reports to the command (through CGBI), scheduling the crew for required readiness exams and procedures as needed, and informing the command when a given crew member or department fails to cooperate with the IDHS's efforts to comply with readiness requirements. The IDHS shall also maintain a tracking system to include all return appointments requested by physicians or dentists from outside referrals requested by the command.

(7) Ensure supplies, materials and equipment necessary to carry out the mission of the Health Services Department are obtained and maintained in sufficient quantity and condition to support the unit mission and operation.

(8) Health Services Department administration, maintenance, and security of health records. Maintain health records as required by Chapter 4 of this Manual. Ensure that all treatment records and/or consults from outside referrals are obtained and placed in the health record. In addition, ensure that each patient is notified of all physical exams, consultations, and diagnostic tests (e.g., pap smears, mammograms,

biopsies, x-rays, etc.) performed at any facility prior to filing in the health record. Maintain the security and confidentiality of all medical/dental records, databases and any other protected health information.

(9) Strict adherence to Chapter 2 of this Manual which contains information about general and specific duties of the HS serving independently, including all required training in compliance with HIPAA privacy and security.

(10) Other duties as assigned by the CO. In accordance with Paragraph 7-5-4, United States Coast Guard Regulations 1992, COMDTINST M5000.3 (series), HS may not be detailed to perform combatant duties in their own defense or protection of the wounded and sick in their charge, which are not prohibited by the Geneva Conventions. However, under routine situations; HSs who bear arms forfeit the special protections for medical personnel afforded by the Geneva Convention.

d. <u>Chain Of Command</u>. The IDHS will report directly to the Executive Officer (XO).

e. <u>Operation of the Health Services Department</u>. The IDHS is tasked with a wide variety and high volume of duties and responsibilities. This section sets forth policy and guidelines designed to assist the IDHS in carrying out assigned duties and responsibilities.

(1) <u>Health Services Department Standard Operating Procedure</u>. In order to successfully manage the Health Services Department the IDHS must use time management and organizational skills and tools. One such tool is a written Standard Operating Procedure (SOP) for the Health Services Department. The SOP will govern the activity of the IDHS and has as its guiding precept the goals and missions of the unit. The SOP will be developed in consultation with the Designated Medical Officer Advisor (DMOA) and submitted in written form to the CO for approval via the chain of command. In addition, the SOP will be reviewed at least annually by the IDHS, DMOA, XO and CO. The approved SOP will be kept in the Health Services Department for easy referral. Copies of pertinent sections will be posted as appropriate. The SOP will include:

(a) A copy of the IDHS's letter of assumption of duties as Health Services Department Representative.

(b) A written daily schedule of events for both underway and inport periods.

(c) Copies of all letters of designation, assignment, and authority that directly impact upon the IDHS or Health Services Department. Examples include those granting "By direction" authority, designation as working Narcotics and Controlled Substances custodian, and assignment of a DMOA.

(d) A copy of the unit's organizational structure. This document will show graphically the IDHS's chain of command.

(e) A listing of duties and responsibilities assigned to the IDHS and the frequency that they are to be carried out. The listing will include both primary and collateral assigned duties.

(f) A listing of all required reports, the format required for submission, the frequency or date required, required routing and required "copy addressees". Incorporation of this information in tabular format provides a quick and easy guide for reference purposes.

(g) A water bill, for the safe handling of potable water.

(h) A unit instruction or SOP for the management of rape or sexual assault cases. The document must provide policy for the Health Services Department action in such cases, names of organizations, points of contact and telephone numbers for local resources as well as contact information for agencies and facilities which must be notified. CGIS must be notified for all unrestricted reports of alleged rape or sexual assault. It must contain a prearranged mechanism for timely completion of a physical examination by a **Sexual Assault Medical Forensic Examiner (SAMFE) or Sexual Assault Nurse Examiner (SANE)** for the purpose of evidence gathering that meets requirements of all applicable law enforcement agencies. Additionally, it must define limitations that will exist if the unit is underway at the time the incident occurs. It must contain directions on how to complete a Victim Reporting Preference Statement, Form CG-6095. **Additionally, it must define the unrestricted and restricted reporting procedures as outlined in the Sexual Assault Prevention and Response (SAPR) Program, COMDTINST M1754.10 (series).**

(i) A unit instruction or SOP for the management of suicide threat or attempt. The document must provide policy for Health Services Department action in such cases, names of organizations, points of contact and telephone numbers for local resources, contact information for agencies and facilities which must be notified as well as a listing of required information, reports or actions.

(j) A unit instruction or SOP action required in the event of family violence. The document must provide policy for Health Services Department action in such cases, names of organizations, points of contact and telephone numbers for local resources, contact information for agencies and facilities which must be notified as well as a listing of required information, reports or actions.

(2) Other Necessary Documents. The IDHS is an integral part of many unit activities and various unit bills and doctrines require specific action by the IDHS. Since these are changed frequently, incorporation of Health Services Department responsibilities contained in these various documents into the Health Services Department SOP is not recommended. Applicable portions should be kept in the Health Services Department for

quick reference, however. These include:

(a) A battle doctrine for the unit.

(b) Portions of the unit mass casualty bill pertaining to Health Services Department responsibility.

(c) Portions of the unit general emergency bill pertaining to Health Services Department responsibility.

(d) Portions of the unit man overboard bill pertaining to Health Services Department responsibility.

(e) Portions of the unit replenishment at sea, special sea detail, flight quarters and bomb threat bills pertaining to Health Services Department responsibility.

f. Departure from the Daily Schedule of Events. The day-to-day operation of the Health Services Department is complex and impacted by the operational needs of the unit. Of necessity, it will change when events of higher priority or concern occur. If deviation from the daily schedule of events is required, notification of the XO (IDHS's Division Officer) will be made at the earliest opportunity. When deviation from daily schedule of events occurs frequently, the daily schedule of events will be reviewed and if necessary, changed. Any changes will be incorporated into the Health Services Department SOP and approved by the Commanding Officer.

g. Relief and Assumption of Duties as the IDHS. Proper documentation of the status of the Health Services Department, the condition of its equipment, stores, and records is required at the time of relief and assumption of the duties and responsibilities as the IDHS. This must be completed in order to adequately ascertain the state of operational medical readiness of the health services department and advise the command. Operational readiness refers to the immediate ability to meet all health care demands within the unit's capabilities. The process is complex and requires both the incoming and outgoing IDHS to jointly perform the following:

(1) A complete inventory of all medical stores, spaces, and equipment, including durable medical equipment. Obtain the unit Health Services Allowance List and inspect the inventory of all health services department equipment, supplies, and publications. Initiate action for repair, survey, or replenishment of equipment, supplies, and publications. Verify inventory records and check all logs. Report any discrepancies to the local command without delay. Amplification of requirements and procedures is contained in Chapters 8 and 10 of this Manual. The Health Services Allowance List Afloat, COMDTINST M6700.6 (series) provides a listing of supplies and the equipment required by each class of vessel.

(a) A controlled substances inventory must be current. Use direction provided in Chapter 10 of this Manual.

(b) A complete inventory of all unit property in custody of the Health

Services Department shall be completed.

(2) A review of ongoing actions affecting the status of Health Services, e.g., outstanding requisitions, survey or repairs, and proper documentation of all such transactions.

(3) A review of the Health Services Department SOP.

(4) A review of the most recent HSWL SC Quality Assurance Assistance Survey for the unit. A copy of the survey annotated with any finding of incomplete or uncorrected discrepancies will be included as an enclosure to the letter of relief.

(5) A review of all health records for completeness, accuracy, privacy and security. Check health records against the personnel roster. Any missing records should be accounted for or requested from previous duty stations. If records cannot be accounted for within one month's time, open a new health record. Check health records for completeness, and if not current, obtain and enter all missing information to the fullest extent possible. (See Chapter 4 of this Manual for further instructions pertaining to health records).

(6) A review of the most recent Tailored Annual Cutter Training evaluation. Paragraph 4 of this section provides the outline for the training program.

(7) A complete health, safety and sanitation inspection of the vessel, to include status of potable water systems (records of bacteriological, halogen content and pH testing), food stores inspections, and berthing and habitability of living and berthing spaces.

h. Letter of Relief and Assumption of Duties. Upon completion of the Health Services Department review a Coast Guard memorandum will be prepared and submitted by the oncoming IDHS via the chain of command and will advise the Commanding Officer of the status of the Health Services Department. A copy of the letter will be forwarded to the HSWL SC Senior IDHS Coordinator. The letter of Relief and Assumption of Duties will provide the following:

(1) Date of assumption of duties. A statement shall be signed by the oncoming IDHS, that the duties and responsibilities of the IDHS have been assumed; and that a thorough review of the Health Services Department has been conducted. Any discrepancies of material or record keeping will be annotated on a copy of the unit's most recent HSWL SC Quality Assurance site survey and submitted as an enclosure to the letter of Relief and Assumption of Duties as IDHS for the vessel.

(2) Any discrepancies noted upon relief will be handled as a matter of individual command prerogative. Responsibility for correction, adjustment of account or inventory records, action required to replace missing items, as well as any necessary disciplinary action will be determined by the command. The district SIDHS shall be consulted for appropriate guidance.

(3) For cases in which no on site relief occurs, all of the preceding action will be completed. The supply officer of the unit will participate as intermediary between outgoing and incoming IDHS. District SIDHS shall be consulted for additional assistance during relief process.

i. Actions upon Proper Relief. Upon assumption of duties as the unit's IDHS, one of the first tasks to complete is a thorough review of all SOPs and department instructions. Check the references; make contact with any listed points of contact (especially with the DMOA). If possible, make visits and introductions in person. Find out how each system works and how it is accessed.

3. Providing Health Care Afloat. Provision of health care is the most challenging and rewarding duty of an IDHS. An IDHS bears a tremendous responsibility, which can never be taken lightly. This section is intended to provide a brief summary of the various facets of providing medical care afloat.

a. Designated Medical Officer Advisor (DMOA). All IDHS shall be assigned a DMOA in accordance with Chapter 1 of this Manual. Good communication between all IDHSs and their DMOA can prevent problems affecting health care delivery to the crew. All IDHSs will schedule a visit with the DMOA as soon as is practical after reporting aboard. This visit will normally be scheduled for a period of at least two weeks. The purpose of the visit is to allow first-hand communication of expectations, support facility requirements, allow for direct oversight of IDHS rendered clinical care, and any unique needs or concerns. Open communication can be maintained through regular visits when practical, or at minimum, regular telephone calls. With regard to provision of direct care, the IDHS will seek DMOA (or surrogate's) advice whenever there are questions about a patient's condition or when the following conditions exist:

(1) Return to sick call before assigned follow-up because of failure to improve or condition has deteriorated.

(2) Member cannot return to full duty status after 72 hours duration because of unresolved illness.

NOTE: The IDHS shall contact the Flight Surgeon on call through the closest Coast Guard Command Center when any of the following emergency conditions exist:

(1) Fever of unknown origin of 102 degrees Fahrenheit or higher (when taken orally) persisting for 48 hours.

(2) Fever of 103 degrees Fahrenheit or higher (when taken orally).

(3) Unexplained pulse rate above 120 beats per minute.

(4) Unexplained respiratory rate above 28 breaths per minute or less than 12 breaths per minute.

(5) Psychosis or Depression with suicidal thoughts.

(6) Change in mental status or level of consciousness.

(7) Chest pain or arrhythmia.

(8) Unexplained shortness of breath.

(9) Rape or sexual assault.

(10) Any condition threatening life or limb.

b. Gender Considerations. Chapter 1 Section B of this Manual provides specific direction for health services technicians about patient privacy, same gender attendant requirements, and examination restrictions.

c. Avoiding Common Problems. Scheduling and obtaining the routine medical care needed by crewmembers during short inport periods can tax the organizational skills of even the most experienced IDHS. There are, however, actions that the IDHS can take which will enhance the chances of getting the routine appointments needed for all members. Some of these are:

(1) Identify the routine medical and dental needs of the crew well in advance of return to port. The vessel's supporting clinic has an established appointment scheduling procedure within which the IDHS must work whenever operational schedules allow. Provide requests via message (or other written form as appropriate) for appointment scheduling ahead of "appointment schedule opening" for the inport period whenever possible. Request reply by message prior to the vessel's scheduled return to port. When routine medical or dental care is to be made directly to a DOD MTF, the IDHS must determine the facility requirements for referral of patients and follow any local procedures.

(2) Communicate with the vessel's supporting clinic. Visit the supporting clinic, if practical, as soon as possible after return to port. Discuss the crew's medical and dental needs with the clinic supervisor and DMOA (if located at the facility).

(3) Perform as many preliminary tests and as much paperwork as possible before scheduling physicals at the supporting clinic.

(4) Post a listing of appointment dates and times as soon as it becomes available. Provide each division officer and shop chief a listing of the appointments applicable to the division or shop.

(5) Hold members accountable to be at their appointed place and time. Provide feedback to division officers and shop chiefs on any appointment failure. Notify XO of more than one failure.

d. Consultations. During the management of complex or protracted cases, consultations or specialty referral may be necessary. When such services are needed, the IDHS will normally contact a CG clinic or in some cases, a Department of Defense medical treatment facility (DOD MTF). When arranging for a patient to see a Medical Officer at a CG clinic, the IDHS shall ensure that a Chronological Record of Care, Form SF-600 entry is completed using the SOAP format and that an appointment is scheduled. The clinic will normally provide treatment or arrange care if treatment is beyond its scope. When consultations or referral for specialty care are required, the IDHS shall coordinate with the PCM. The IDHS must determine the facility requirements for referral of patients and follow any local procedures. Referrals to a DOD MTF will normally be documented using an Consultation Sheet, Form SF-513, Consultation Sheet or a Referral for Civilian Medical Care, Form DD-2161. The consultation request shall provide a concise history of the condition to be evaluated as well as any pertinent findings and a provisional diagnosis. Chapter 4 Section B of this Manual provides direction on completion of a Consultation Sheet, Form SF-513. The patient should inform their supervisor of all referral appointment dates and times. Whenever possible, provide at least 24 hours notice for changes or cancellations.

e. Medical Evacuation (MEDEVAC) of Injured or Ill Crewmembers. Medical evacuation must be considered when care is needed by a patient to preserve life or limb, provide pain relief beyond capability onboard, or to provide other medical or dental treatment for which delay until the unit's next scheduled port call would provide undue hardship or pain for the patient. The unit's ability to MEDEVAC a patient will be affected by the vessel's current mission, availability of air transport assets, and location. When considering or executing a MEDEVAC:

(1) Keep the XO informed. At first indication that a MEDEVAC may become necessary, notify the XO.

(2) Request, via the XO, communication with the closest Coast Guard command center and request to consult with the Flight Surgeon on call. In addition to a thorough patient presentation, information about the unit's location in relation to medical resources ashore and realistic estimations of time requirements to reach a point that MEDEVAC is possible, must be available. Keep the Flight Surgeon advised of any change in the patient's condition.

(3) Thoroughly document the MEDEVAC process. Ensure that a complete patient record is maintained in the patient's health record. Maintain a complete record of events in the Health Services log. Make entries as events occur.

(4) Keep the patient informed. Explain in as much detail as possible the actions being taken and expected outcome of the actions. As time of departure approaches, describe for the patient what to expect during transport and upon arrival at destination. If a Coast Guard Beneficiary Representative is attached to the medical facility to which the patient is being MEDEVACed, provide this information to the patient.

(5) Ensure that all information about the patient's is current on the Adult Preventive and Chronic Care Flowsheet, Form DD-2766. The Adult Preventive and Chronic Care Flowsheet, Form DD-2766 should

accompany the patient with record of current illness/injury – Chronological Record of Care, Form SF-600. Ensure that information necessary for unit contact and contact of the unit's supporting clinic are provided and easily located by the receiving medical facility. Anticipate the patient's need for personal items, including a valid Armed Forces Identification Card, and ensure these are packaged for transport with the patient. Limit such items to those that are necessary. Encourage the patient to limit cash. Ensure proper medical preparation of the patient for medevac, particularly if to be hosted via litter or basket.

 (6) Notify the unit's supporting clinic and DMOA of the MEDEVAC and any needed assistance for the patient.

 (7) Provide an inpatient hospitalization notification e-mail in accordance with current directives. See Chapter 2 Section A of this Manual.

f. Surgical Procedures. Most routine minor surgical procedures will be delayed until the vessel is in port. Surgical procedures while underway will be limited to only those procedures that are needed in order to return a patient to a fit for full duty status. These procedures include:

 (1) Placing and removing sutures in a wound.

 (2) Incision and drainage.

 (3) Unguinectomy.

 (4) Paring down painful plantar warts.

g. Refusal of Treatment. Medical, dental, and surgical treatment will not be performed on a mentally competent member who does not consent to the recommended procedure except when (with DMOA endorsement):

 (1) Emergency care is required to preserve the life or health of the member.

 (2) Isolation and quarantine of suspected or proven communicable diseases as medically indicated or required by law to ensure proper treatment and protection of the member or others.

h. Motion Sickness. Members that manifest chronic motion sickness, that do not respond to conventional therapy, and are unable to perform their duties as a result, will be considered for administrative separation from active duty as per the Military Separations, COMDTINST M1000.4 (series).

i. Antibiotic Therapy. The IDHS may prescribe and administer antibiotics included on the Health Services Allowance List Afloat. Whenever possible, the IDHS shall consult with his/her DMOA or surrogate for a recommendation or concurrence prior to administering antibiotic therapy.

j. Health Services Treatment Space. The Health Services treatment space will be manned at all times when patients are inside. All items are to be stowed in their proper place and secured. All medical records shall be locked in a cabinet. At no time should the Health Services space be left unlocked when the IDHS is not onboard.

k. Patient Berthing. Some units have facilities for close patient observation or treatment. Absolutely no person other than the sick or injured will be berthed in the Health Services Department. The IDHS may sleep in the Health Services Department when attending an injured or sick patient, but will have a regularly assigned berthing space. Personal gear and clothing are not to be stored in the Health Services Department. The Health Services Department will not be used as berthing spaces for augmented personnel.

l. Not Fit For Sea Duty. Members who are medically, surgically, or orthopedically unfit for sea duty (including wearing a cast or needing to use crutches) and unable to perform their duties will not be placed onboard the vessel. Personnel will either be placed on Limited Duty ashore or on Convalescent Leave.

m. Convalescent Leave/Sick Leave. Convalescent leave/Sick leave is a period of leave not charged against a member's leave account. It can be a recommendation to the command when a patient is Not Fit For Duty (usually for a duration expected to be greater than 72 hours) and whose recovery time can reasonably be expected to improve by freedom from the confines of quarters. It should be considered only when required as an adjunct to patient treatment. The command must evaluate each recommendation. Commands are authorized to grant convalescent leave as outlined in Military Assignments and Authorized Absences, COMDTINST M1000.8 (series). The IDHS shall re-evaluate all patients at the termination of their approved convalescent/sick leave.

n. Controlled Substances. Regulations for the handling, storage, and issue of narcotics and controlled substances are found in Chapter 10 of this Manual. The contents of this section are not intended to contradict the guidance provided there. This section serves to amplify policy provided with respect to medicinal narcotics and controlled substances onboard afloat units.

   (1) Narcotics and controlled substances require special handling. All controlled substances shall be obtained through the unit's collateral duty Regional Pharmacy Executive (RPE).

   (2) The CO will designate the Executive Officer as the controlled substances custodian (CSC). The CSC will follow the accounting procedure provided in Chapter 10 of this Manual. The IDHS will normally be assigned as custodian for narcotics and controlled substances working stock. Such assignment must be made in writing.

   (3) All issues from working stock will be documented with a properly completed, written prescription. All non-emergent care requires contact with a Medical Officer before dispensing any controlled medication. The Medical Officer's orders will be documented on a prescription and in the patient's health record. The words "By verbal order of" will precede the ordering Medical Officer's initials, last name, and time of order and date of order both on the prescription and in the patient's health record. In the event of an emergency, a Medical Officer's order is not needed to

dispense a controlled substance. Once the emergency situation is over or alleviated, the IDHS will contact a Medical Officer and detail the circumstances and the controlled substances that were administered. Upon concurrence by the Medical Officer, the prescription prepared for the patient will be annotated with the words "By concurrence of" the ordering physician's initials, last name, time of concurrence and date of concurrence.

(4) The XO will countersign all prescriptions prepared by the IDHS prior to issue of any controlled substance or narcotic.

(5) Controlled substances stored aboard cutters shall be limited to amounts in the Health Services Allowance List, Afloat, COMDTINST M6700.6 (series) . If the need exists for the unit to carry additional quantities of controlled substances based on use or potential for operational need, a written request signed by the Commanding Officer will be forwarded to the IDHS's DMOA. The request must include nomenclature, quantity, and brief justification.

o. Dental. It is the duty of the IDHS to arrange for the necessary dental examinations of the crew. All personnel should be Class I or Class II prior to deployment and results shall be documented in DENCAS.

(1) All personnel must receive an annual dental exam.

(2) The IDHS will arrange, via e-mail or message, for the large group of dental appointments needed for crewmembers returning from deployment. A signup sheet and announcement to the crewmembers is advised, and early communication with the staff of the dental clinic is recommended in order to allow sufficient time for the scheduling of a large amount of dental visits. Urgent cases obviously are to be scheduled first, regardless of rank or position of the member. Once back in port, active communication with a designated POC in the dental clinic is advised in order to handle cancellations, substitutions and last minute appointment changes. Although it may be time consuming, it is easier to deliver patient reminders the morning of the scheduled appointment than to try and explain a group of no-show crewmembers to a dental officer or XO.

p. Rape or Sexual Assault. All victims of rape or sexual assault must be treated in a professional, compassionate and non-judgmental manner. Examination of rape and sexual assault victims will be limited to only visual examination of any wound or injury and treated according to present standards of care. In all cases, a Medical Officer and CGIS will be contacted for advice. In the event that no Medical Officer is available (underway), an IDHS may conduct the visual examination. A chaperone of the same gender as the patient will be present if such examination is conducted. All aspects of the patient encounter must be carefully documented. Physical examination to gather evidence of rape or sexual assault is strictly prohibited. The unit shall have a SOP for alleged rape and sexual assault. Refer to Sexual Assault Prevention and

Response **(SAPR) Program, COMDTINST M1754.10 (series).**

q. Suicide Prevention. An encounter with a suicidal person is always a deeply emotional event. It is important for the IDHS to act in a caring and professional manner. Early intervention and good communication skills are essential. If suicidal ideation is suspected, it is important to remember:

(1) Take all threats and symptoms seriously. Asking about suicidal thoughts will not "put the idea in the person's head" or increase the risk of suicide. Raising the subject gives permission for open discussion. For any member considering suicide, immediately seek professional help from the nearest MTF or civilian emergency room with facilities appropriate to the situation. At no time should the person be left unattended. Once the patient is safe, contact the servicing Work-Life office for additional help or refer to Suicide Prevention Program, COMDTINST 1734.1 (series).

(2) Actively listen to the patient. Do not argue, judge, attempt to diagnose, or analyze the person's true intentions. It is important to provide a calm, caring, professional demeanor throughout the entire situation. Thoroughly document the patient encounter using the SOAP format.

(3) Arrange for an escort and a driver to transport the patient to the nearest Coast Guard clinic, MTF or civilian emergency room with facilities appropriate to the situation. The unit's SOP for suicide threat or attempt should contain this information for ready use if needed. If underway, then a MEDEVAC must be considered. Contact a Flight Surgeon, the IDHS's DMOA or a Medical Officer familiar with the area of operation for advice on how to handle this patient.

(4) Completion of Applied Suicide Intervention Skills (ASIS) Training is highly recommended. For further information refer to the Suicide Prevention Program, COMDTINST 1734.1 (series).

r. Decedent Affairs. Chapter 5 of this Manual contains guidance about action that the Health Services Department must take when there is a death aboard a Coast Guard unit. Military Casualties and Decedent Affairs, COMDTINST M1770.9 (series) contains further guidance concerning casualties and decedent affairs, as does the Decedent Affairs Guide, COMDTINST M1770.1 (series). It is unlikely that the IDHS will be assigned as the Casualty Assistance Calls Officer (CACO) for the command, but the IDHS will undoubtedly be heavily involved with the process of proper disposition of remains, so familiarity with the information required is helpful. The IDHS should also perform the following:

(1) An entry in the Health Services Log will be made detailing all available information concerning the death.

(2) The health record of the deceased member will be terminated in accordance with Chapter 4 of this Manual.

s. <u>Disposition of Remains</u>. As soon as possible, remains will be transferred to the nearest Military Treatment Facility (MTF) for further disposition. When transfer cannot be accomplished immediately, the remains will be placed into a body pouch and refrigerated at a temperature of 36 to 40 degrees Fahrenheit to prevent decomposition. The space must contain no other items and must be cleaned and disinfected before reuse. Remains will be identified with a waterproof tag, marked with waterproof ink, and affixed with wire ties to the right great toe of the decedent and also to each end of the body pouch. The minimum information needed on each tag includes the full name, SSN and rate or rank of the decedent. Whenever possible, do not remove items attached to the deceased at time of death. Such items may include (for example) IV lines, needles, AED pads, ET tubes, lengths of cord or line, etc. These may be important during an autopsy. In the event of a mishap, notify the Duty Flight Surgeon and DMOA to ensure attendance at the post-mortem examination and Mishap Analysis. Additionally, do not discard or launder clothing of the deceased. These items are sometimes important to surviving family members and in some cultures is part of the mourning process for the deceased. This is a cultural consideration but should be a part of the decision process.

t. <u>Physical Disability Evaluation System</u>. The medical board process is detailed in Military Casualties and Decedent Affairs, COMDTINST M1770.9 (series) and the Physical Disability Evaluation Manual, COMDTINST M1850.2 (series).

4. <u>Training</u>. The purpose of training provided to the crew of an afloat unit include: assurance that crewmembers are able to provide aid for themselves and their shipmates in an emergency or a combat situation and to promote the general health and well being of the crew. To this end, a written Health Services Department Training Plan will be prepared and submitted to the unit training officer for incorporation into the unit training plan and the SIDHS for quality assurance review.

a. <u>Health Services Department Training Plan</u>. A plan for training of the crew will be established. The plan will be established in written form and kept on file. It will be based on a minimum 12 month cycle and be included in the cutter training schedule. At a minimum, the following training will be given annually:

(1) Basic first aid.

(2) Shock, hemorrhage control, and bandaging.

(3) Airway management and assisted ventilation.

(4) Route to battle dressing stations (BDS) and use of items in first aid kits gunbags and boxes.

(5) Personal and dental hygiene.

(6) STI/HIV prevention.

(7) Heat and cold stress programs, including hypothermia.

(8) Respiratory protection program.

(9) Hearing conservation.

(10) Sight conservation.

(11) Blood borne pathogens.

b. Documentation of Training. Documentation of the training is a Tailored Annual Cutter Training requirement as well as a requirement of several Coast Guard programs. The rule of thumb to remember is "If it isn't written down, it didn't happen." An outline must be prepared and kept on file for all training topics presented and a training log maintained for all training provided. The training log will contain a record of all HS training given to the crew, stretcher-bearers, and HSs. It will contain the following information:

(1) Date.

(2) Topic.

(3) Duration.

(4) Group or department receiving the training.

(5) Instructor's name.

(6) Names (signatures of those present) of members trained.

c. Training Format. Training will normally be presented in either lecture format or demonstration and practical application. Lecture format presentations should be limited to 15 to 20 minutes and demonstrations and practical application should not exceed 1 hour. Practical application must be of high priority in training the crew and stretcher-bearers in first aid, casualty evaluation, treatment, reports to damage control central, and transporting casualties to battle dressing stations. There is no substitute for "hands on" practice in developing effective first aid and patient transport skills.

d. Departmental Training. Specific training not applicable to the entire crew, but appropriate to individual departments, should be incorporated into the Health Services Training Plan. Such departmental training is normally needed because of workplace exposure to potential health hazards. Training subjects appropriate to various departments are listed in the following subparagraphs. The list is not all inclusive. It is provided as a guideline.

(1) Weapons department:

(a) Hearing conservation.

(b) Heat stress (ship's laundry personnel).

(c) Respiratory protection.

(d) Basic life support (fire control personnel).

        (e) Review of prevention and treatment of electric shock casualties.

        (f) Eyesight protection.

        (g) Self-Aid/Buddy-Aid

    (2) Engineering department:

        (a) Hearing conservation.

        (b) Potable water.

        (c) Heat stress.

        (d) Respiratory protection.

        (e) Eyesight protection.

        (f) Hazards associated with human waste.

    (3) Supply department:

        (a) Food service sanitation (food service personnel).

        (b) Heat stress (scullery personnel).

        (c) Injury Prevention.

    (4) Operations department:

        (a) Basic life support (electronics shop personnel).

        (b) Review of prevention and treatment of burns, electric shock and hemorrhage.

    (5) Deck department:

        (a) Eyesight protection.

        (b) Hearing conservation.

        (c) Heat stress.

        (d) Respiratory protection.

e. <u>Drills</u>. Drills are a necessary part of unit training. Drills help to reinforce performance of skills and actions that must be completed during stressful or potentially dangerous situations. Drills that have close relation to health and safety of the crew will be incorporated into the Health Services Department Training Plan. The cutter training board should integrate Health Services Department Training Plan drills into the unit's training schedule.

    (1) The following drills will be conducted semi-annually:

        (a) Battle Dressing Station.

        (b) Personnel casualty transportation.

        (c) Mass casualty.

(2) The following drills, at minimum, will be conducted quarterly:

    (a) Compound fracture.

    (b) Sucking chest wound.

    (c) Abdominal wounds.

    (d) Amputation.

    (e) Facial wounds.

    (f) Electrical shock.

    (g) Smoke inhalation.

    (h) Casualty transport.

    (i) SA/BA

f. Training and Assignment of Stretcher-Bearers. No less than four stretcher-bearers will be assigned to the Primary Battle Dressing station (BDS). The training for stretcher-bearers will include all subjects given to the crew with emphasis on basic first aid, casualty evacuation, triage, use of all stretcher types maintained onboard the unit, casualty carrying methods, setup and organization and basic life support. Stretcher-bearers must also complete the advanced first aid portion of the Damage Control Personnel Qualification Standards (DC PQS).

g. Training for the IDHS. Careful study, practice, and concentration on all facets of the Health Services Technician are necessary to prepare an HS to be successful as an IDHS. In addition to the requirements of the rating, successful completion of certain training and "C" schools are required as per Cutter Training and Qualification Manual, COMDTINST M3502.4 (series) These are:

(1) Coast Guard Independent Duty Health Services Technician, Air Force Medical Services Craftsman or Navy Surface Forces Independent Duty Technician.

(2) Coast Guard Introduction to Environmental Health or Navy Basic Shipboard Series. (Note: This is not required for graduates of Navy Surface Forces Independent Duty Technician or Independent Duty Health Services Technician School).

(3) Emergency Medical Technician. IDHS assigned to a floating unit are required to maintain currency with the National Registry of Emergency Medical Technicians (NREMT) at the EMT level. Short Term Training Requests are to be completed in accordance with the Training and Education Manual, COMDTINST M1500.10 (series) and forwarded to Commandant (CG-1121). Funding will be provided by Commandant (CG-11). See the Emergency Medical Services Manual, COMDTINST M16135.4 (series) for additional information.

(4) Instructor courses (Must maintain current certification in) CPR, BLS, AED and First Aid.

(5) <u>Field Management of Chemical and Biological Casualties</u>. The Field Management of Chemical and Biological Casualties Course (FCBC) is conducted by the US Army Medical Research Institute of Chemical Defense (USAMRICD) at Aberdeen Proving Ground, Maryland. Classroom instruction, laboratory and field exercises prepare graduates to become trainers in the first echelon management of chemical and biological agent casualties. This course is required per Cutter Training and Qualification Manual, COMDTINST M3502.4 (series).

h. <u>IDHS Initial Certification</u>. All newly assigned IDHSs will participate in an orientation and certification program at their supporting clinic. Initial orientation must be completed within 60 days of reporting in to the new unit. If due to operational commitments the orientation and certification can not be completed within 60 days of reporting, a waiver request must be sent in memo format to the HSWL RP SIDHS Team Leader. If the unit is unable to fund the TDY, the IDHS shall request funding from their HSWL RP SIDHS. Initial orientation and certification is estimated to take 2 weeks. During this time, the IDHS will:

(1) Work with his/her DMOA to complete the IDHS Operational Integration, Form CG-6000-4.

(2) See a minimum of 12 patients

(3) Perform a focused exam on each of the body's systems while using the DMOA as a guide and evaluator.

(4) Discuss with his/her DMOA the notification procedures for the dispensing of scheduled drugs, administration of emergency medications and antibiotics.

(5) Solicit documented feedback from the DMOA and work to improve any areas where required.

(6) Perform a minimum of 4 clinical hours with a dental preceptor.

(7) Solicit documented feedback from the dental preceptor and work to improve any areas where required.

(8) Demonstrate a verbal understanding of management of acute dental problems to include dental abscess, periodontal disease, temporary fillings, fractured teeth, etc.

(9) Demonstrate documentation requirements for dental problems.

i. <u>IDHS Annual Sustainment Training Requirements</u>. Every 12 months, the IDHS must complete the following task:

(1) <u>See a minimum of 48 patients/year</u>. The IDHS shall solicit feedback from his/her DMOA on the patients treated over the last year.

(2) Work with his/her DMOA to complete the IDHS Operational Integration, Form CG-6000-4.

(3) Instruct at least one BLS certification class. Submit training roster to the district SIDHS.

(4) Review all CEUs acquired over the last year in order to maintain EMT certification with his/her DMOA.

j. <u>Training for the Junior HS Aboard Cutters</u>. If a junior HS is assigned to a cutter TAD, he/she is considered an apprentice for training purposes. The cutter HSC is responsible for the training and mentorship of the junior HS. While assigned, the junior HS shall accomplish the following training requirements:

(1) Completion of Enlisted Performance Quals for next paygrade.

(2) While inport, attend weekly training sessions at supporting CG Clinic. This shall include spending clinical time working with their assigned DMOA. If cutter is not co-located with their DMOA Clinic, the junior HS should attend formal clinical training at a local MTF if available.

(3) Submit 100% of their record entries to the HSC for quality assurance review and training opportunities. The HSC must provide feedback to the junior HS with a copy to the district SIDHS for filing.

5. <u>Supply and Logistics</u>.

a. <u>Custody of Health Services Equipment and Material</u>. As directed by the Commanding Officer, the IDHS is responsible and accountable for the health services material onboard the cutter. As such, the IDHS is the custodian of all health service equipment and material. The custodian will not permit waste or abuse of supplies or equipment and will use techniques such as stock rotation, planned replacement and preventive maintenance to minimize waste of resources.

b. <u>Inventory</u>. An accurate record of medical stores and equipment must be maintained. The inventory of medical stores, spaces and equipment will be prepared using the NAVSUP-1114, Stock Record Card Afloat or in line item form (computerized database is an approved and preferred alternative if all necessary information is captured) and include

(1) Quantity and shelf-life of each item currently on board.

(2) Balance on hand, high-level, low-level (reorder point for each item).

(3) Manufacturer, lot number and expiration date (pharmaceuticals).

(4) Quantity placed on order, date received.

c. <u>Unit Property</u>. Unit property in Health Services Department custody must also be safeguarded and accounted for. The unit property custodian should be contacted before transfer or destruction of such property.

d. <u>Funding and Account Record Keeping</u>. Funds used to purchase supplies and equipment and to pay for the various expenses of operating the unit are broken down into Allotment Fund Control (AFC) expenditure categories. This method allows for efficient budgeting and accounting. Fund categories generally used by an IDHS fall within the AFC subhead 30 or 57 expenditure categories.

   (1) AFC-30 is a general ship fund used by the supply department to purchase generally needed operating supplies and services. Examples include pens, paper, books, training aids, etc. AFC-30 funding can be used to pay for Health Services Department supplies and equipment not obtainable through Defense Supply Center Philadelphia Prime Vendor Program (via the unit's supporting clinic) or the major medical equipment request process (see Chapters 6 and 8 of this Manual). Restrictions exist on what may be purchased with AFC-30 funds. Specific questions can be answered by unit supply personnel.

   (2) AFC-57 is a funding category used to purchase health care related supplies and equipment, and to pay for health care. AFC-57 funds are distributed to the HSWL SC for further distribution to the units within their areas of responsibility with HS's assigned.

   (3) With the full implementation of the Prime Vendor programs for Pharmaceuticals and for Medical and Surgical Supplies, AFC-57 fund allocations will be made to the Prime Vendor ordering point assigned for the unit.

   (4) All 5211 requests submitted by the IDHS shall be validated by the RP SIDHS then forwarded to HSWL SC SIDHS for approval and purchase.

e. Budgets and Budgeting. In general, IDHSs do not need to plan and submit an AFC-57 budget request because medical supplies and equipment funding are controlled by the HSWL SC and Prime Vendor ordering points. If additional AFC-57 resource needs are anticipated, the IDHS's supporting clinic should be contacted for direction on how the resources are to be requested. The budget build process does have value for the IDHS however. AFC-30 funds will need to be planned for and requested and medical equipment in need of planned replacement must be identified and a Coast Guard Health Care Equipment Request, Form CG-5211 submitted. The budget build process is a good way to handle these needs. AFC-30 fund budget planning is relatively straight forward, although it can be time consuming. AFC-30 expenditures for Health Services should be broken into general use categories. Examples of categories are books and publications, non-consumable goods and services such as hydro testing and replacement of oxygen cylinders, annual calibration of heat stress meters, and travel for continuing education. Budgeting categories can be as simple or complicated as the IDHS desires to make it. Once categories have been established, a ledger for the Health Services Department should be "opened" and the expenditure categories entered into it. The use of a "spreadsheet" program is an efficient way to keep an accounting record, but a ledger book works just as well. Attention to detail is the key. In general, a system using four to five categories works well.

(1) In preparing a budget for the upcoming year, it is important to look back over what was purchased in the previous year. To do this, collect all records of AFC 30 orders and expenditures. Review each line item and record the amount spent into the appropriate budget category. The following is a timeline on how to prepare a budget.

March	Look back process. Review amount of funds spent over the first two quarters of the fiscal year as well as spending patterns for the previous fiscal year. Note general categories on which funds were spent and in which quarter items were ordered. This will allow projection of quarterly funding needs into the upcoming year.
April/May	Review status of the Health Services Department medical library and determine which texts and references must be updated.
	Review status of HS certifications and continuing medical education. Funding for training, conferences or seminars not normally funded by AFC 56 funds must be budgeted for as AFC 30 budget line items.
	Review preventive maintenance records and include cost projections in AFC 30 budget. Prepare and submit any Coast Guard Health Care Equipment Request, Form CG-5211 for medical equipment to be replaced.
	Seek guidance from XO on known or planned activities outside normal operations. An example is a yard period (which will require higher than normal supplies of various personal protective equipment (PPE)) or extended deployments in which normal supply is difficult.
June	Submit finalized budget proposal through chain of command. AFC 30 budget information will be added to the unit budget. Be prepared to "defend" the budget request submitted. Documentation of the data gathering process and retrieval of the raw data used to justify the funding requested will likely be required. AFC 56 funds requests will be consolidated by the command and forwarded to the unit's district, HSWL SC or Area commander, as appropriate.

Table 9-A-1

(2) Careful stewardship, good record keeping and accounting make existing funding and justification for increased funding levels easier.

f. Obtaining Pharmaceuticals, Medical and Surgical Supplies. Chapter 8 of this Manual provides policy applicable to the management of Health Services supplies. Prime Vendor programs for both Pharmaceuticals and Medical/Surgical Supplies have been established and it is through these programs that essentially all pharmaceuticals and supplies will be obtained. From an "afloat" perspective important aspects of the program include:

(1) Each afloat unit has been assigned a Prime Vendor ordering point for Pharmaceuticals and for Medical/Surgical Supplies. The HSWL SC assigns the POCs and periodically updates the information. The Prime Vendor ordering point may be different for each of the programs.

(2) Funding for both Prime Vendor for Pharmaceuticals and Prime Vendor for Medical/Surgical Supplies is provided to the assigned Prime Vendor ordering point by the HSWL SC. Internal accounting procedures vary among Prime Vendor ordering points. Some have established individual "accounts" for the units they are responsible for while others manage funds from a central account. Regardless of the accounting method used by the Prime Vendor ordering point, the IDHS must establish and maintain a system to track expenditures.

(3) Prime Vendor ordering points establish pharmaceutical and medical/surgical supply ordering procedures for their assigned units. Pharmaceutical and medical supply items ordered will be those required by the Health Services Allowance List (HSAL) in quantities required for the unit type. Deviation from the HSAL requirements will normally occur only after justification of the need is made by the IDHS to the DMOA for the unit. It will be made in writing and kept on file for review during a HSWL SC site surveys.

g. Health Services Supporting Clinic. The supporting clinic for a vessel is the IDHS's partner in providing health care for the vessel's crew. Local agreements and resources may be available to allow the supporting clinic to provide a broader range of services to the IDHS and the vessel's crew but at a minimum, the following will be provided.

(1) All supplies and equipment (under $500.00) listed in the HSAL for the class of vessel and on the HS Core Formulary. The unit no longer receives AFC-57 funding for the operation of the Health Services Department. These funds are provided instead to the vessel's supporting clinic with the intent that the supporting clinic will provide all required items for the IDHS to operate the Health Services Department.

(2) Assign to the IDHS a DMOA in writing. The DMOA shall be available for questions about patient care, as well as completing record reviews quarterly.

(3) Perform medical boards for the IDHS unit as necessary.

(4) Provide a resource for advice and support in all administrative areas of health care provision to include medical administration, physical examination review (within the approving authority of the Health Services Administrator), health benefits, medical billing and bill payment processing assistance, dental care pharmacy administration, supply and logistics, bio-medical waste management, IDHS continuing education, and quality assurance support. Any services provided at the clinic shall be extended to the IDHS to the maximum extent possible.

h. Preventive Maintenance of Health Services Equipment. Chapter 8 of this Manual details the preventive maintenance program for Health Services equipment. Chapters 1 and 2 of the Health Services Allowance List Afloat, COMDTINST M6700.6 (series) provide guidance on the maintenance of specific items carried onboard ship (i.e. gunbags, portable medical lockers, stokes litter, etc.). An important part of medical readiness is a program of preventive maintenance and planned equipment replacement. Repair and routine replacement part costs should be recorded on a locally generated form or side B of Medical/Dental Equipment Maintenance Record, Form NAVMED 6700-3CG. Capture of this data will allow more accurate forecasting of AFC-57 funding needs for preventive maintenance.

i. Replacement of Health Care Equipment. Chapter 8 of this Manual provides direction on how to obtain replacement of health care equipment. An effectively managed planned equipment replacement program minimizes repair costs and avoids loss of critical equipment at unscheduled times. Additionally, used but still serviceable equipment can be used by other facilities by "turn-in and reissue" through the Defense Reutilization Management Office (DRMO). At least annually, normally during the budgeting process, review the preventive maintenance costs for each piece of health care equipment. When repair and maintenance costs for the year exceed 50 percent of the current replacement cost of the equipment, then a From CG-5211, U. S. Coast Guard Health Care Equipment Request should be submitted to the HSWL SC requesting replacement.

j. Disposal of Unserviceable or Outdated Medical Material.

(1) Equipment and Supplies. The Property Management Manual, COMDTINST M4500.5 (series) provides guidance on when a formal survey is required. In general, a formal survey is not required except when equipment has been lost or stolen. If uncertain about whether or not a formal survey should be done, the unit's supply officer should be consulted.

(2) Pharmaceuticals and Medicinals. Destruction of pharmaceuticals and medicinals will rarely be required. Chapter 8.C. of this Manual directs that materials will not be disposed of at sea, but prepared for destruction and held in a secure area until the vessel's return to port where they can be disposed of in accordance with federal, state and local laws.

(a) Prime Vendors provide a partial credit for some materials returned to them. IDHSs and supporting clinics will establish local policy for transfer of expired or short shelf-life pharmaceuticals. A transfer and replacement of pharmaceuticals within 6 months of expiration should be made with the supporting clinic to minimize waste.

(b) If destruction is required, it will be accomplished in a well-ventilated area. Liquid substances present potential exposure through splash back. At a minimum, splash proof goggles and neoprene rubber gloves will be worn when working with liquid substances that may be absorbed through the skin. The wearing of protective equipment such as a splash apron is also encouraged. Thorough hand washing after the destruction process must be accomplished. Medical material must be disposed of in a manner so as to ensure that the material is rendered non-recoverable for use and harmless to the environment. Destruction must be complete, to preclude the use of any portion of a pharmaceutical. Chapter 8. C. of this Manual provides detailed information about destruction and disposal of unsuitable medications.

k. <u>Disposal of Medical Waste</u>. Federal regulation defines how medical waste must be stored and disposed of, and the records that must be kept to document the storage and disposal. The information in the following paragraphs is provided as a general explanation of program requirements rather than an in-depth instruction on handling of medical waste. Medical waste must be classified in one of two categories: potentially infectious or non-infectious waste. In depth guidance about storage, disposal and required record keeping for medical waste can be found in Chapter 13 of this Manual, in Quality Improvement Implementation Guide (QIIG) 16, and in Chapter 5 of the Safety and Environmental Health Manual, COMDTINST M5100.47 (series). An additional source of information is the unit's hazardous material control officer. In general, the disposal and record keeping requirements for the waste depend on the waste category and are:

(1) Potentially infectious waste is defined as an agent that may contain pathogens that may cause disease in a susceptible host. Used needles, scalpel blades, ("sharps"), syringes, soiled dressings, sponges, drapes and surgical gloves will generate the majority of potentially infectious waste. Potentially infectious waste (other than sharps) will be double bagged in biohazard bags, autoclaved if possible and stored in a secure area until disposed of ashore.

(2) Used sharps will be collected in an approved "sharps" container and retained on board for disposal ashore. "Sharps" will not be clipped. Needles will not be recapped.

(3) An adequate supply of storage and disposal material (containers, bags, etc.), must be maintained on board to ensure availability even on a long or unexpected deployment.

(4) A medical bio-hazardous waste log must be establish and maintained,

and must be kept on file for a period of 5 years. A medical bio-hazardous waste log must include the following information:

(a) Date of entry.

(b) Type of waste.

(c) Amount (in weight or volume).

(d) Storage location.

(e) Method of disposal.

(f) Identification number (if required by the state regulating authority). If such a number is required, the authority will provide it.

(5) Non-infectious waste includes disposable medical supplies that do not fall into hazardous waste. Non-infectious waste will be treated as general waste and does not require autoclaving or special handling. It should be placed into an appropriate receptacle and discarded with other general waste.

6. <u>Health Services Department Administration.</u>

a. <u>Required Reports, Logs, and Records.</u> Clear, accurate record keeping is of paramount importance for the IDHS. The quality of care provided to the unit's crew is reflected in the thoroughness of record and log entries completed by the IDHS. During compliance inspections, Tailored Annual Cutter Training and customer assistance visits, the IDHS and the unit will be evaluated at least in part on the accuracy and completeness of the reports and records created and maintained by the IDHS. The following records will be maintained in the Health Services Department. They will be in book/log form and in sufficient detail to serve as a complete and historical record for actions, incidents and data.

(1) <u>Health Services Log.</u> A Health Services Department log will be maintained by the IDHS. This log is a legal document. Entries will be clearly written in a concise, professional manner. The log may be either hand written or prepared using a standard workstation but must be kept on file in "hard copy" form. It is used to document the daily operation of the Health Services Department. At a minimum, it will contain the names of all individuals reporting to sickcall for treatment, inspections, inventories conducted, and the results of potable water testing. The log will be signed daily by the IDHS. It is worth noting that the Health Services Log will provide the information used in the Binnacle List (see required reports in this Chapter and Chapter 4 of this Manual), so a complete record containing information required in the binnacle list as well as other information of interest will streamline preparation of the report. All protected health information in the log must be kept private and secure in compliance with HIPAA.

(a) <u>Training Log.</u> See "Training" in this Chapter.

(b) <u>Potable Water Quality Log</u>. This log will document the date, location and results of free available Chlorine residual or Bromine testing and bacteriological testing. Such logs will be maintained in chronological order, record the date and time of test, type of test, collection site, and results of testing. Potable water quality logs must be kept onboard for 2 years. A sample Potable Water Quality Log is available for local reproduction in Chapter 1, Appendix 1.A of the Water Supply and Wastewater Disposal Manual, COMDTINST M6240.5 (series).

(c) <u>Biohazard Waste Log</u>. This log will contain information as provided in Chapter 13 of this Manual.

(d) <u>Health Records</u>. Health records will be maintained and checked for accuracy as outlined in Chapter 4 of this Manual. A Health Record Receipt, Form NAVMED 6150-7 will be used whenever a Health Record leaves the custody of the IDHS. A quarterly check using the unit's alpha roster will ensure that any oversight is identified in a reasonably timely manner. All records checked out and not returned shall be reported to the command. In the event of Abandon Ship, make necessary arrangements to retrieve health records, if possible. Retrieving health records will be secondary to treating and evacuating casualties.

(2) <u>Required Reports</u>. Numerous reports are required at various intervals. A brief explanation along with a reference is provided for those not mentioned elsewhere in this chapter. Additionally, the information is provided in tabular format at the end of this section.

(a) <u>Binnacle List</u>. The binnacle list is normally a part of the Health Services Department Log. It is a listing of the names of the members provided treatment and the duty status determination resulting from the treatment. The list must be kept daily and submitted to the command for review as directed by the CO. It is normally reviewed each week by the XO and signed by the CO. A copy of the binnacle list should also be routed to the DMOA simultaneously.

(b) <u>Injury Reports</u>. See Paragraph 8. of this Section.

(c) <u>Disease Alert Reports</u>. See Chapter 7-B. of this Manual for requirements.

(d) <u>Inpatient Hospitalization Report</u>. See Chapter 2-A. of this Manual.

(e) <u>Food Service Sanitation Inspection Report</u>. See the Food Service Sanitation Manual, COMDTINST M6240.4 (series) and Paragraph 10-a-(2) of this Chapter.

(f) <u>Potable Water Quality Discrepancy Report</u>. Required by Chapter 1-K.6 of the Water Supply and Wastewater Disposal Manual, COMDTINST M6240.5 (series) when potable water quality fails to meet requirements or is suspect.

(g) <u>Readiness Report</u>. The IDHS will assist the command in ensuring the medical and dental readiness for the personnel in their command by providing monthly Medical and Dental Readiness reports to the command.

Table 9-A-2

Reports Required Weekly

Report Name	Format or Form Required	Reference	Frequency or Date
Binnacle List	locally designed form	COMDTINST M6000.1 (series) Chap 1. Section B.	Compiled daily, submitted weekly (or as directed by command).
Food Service Establishment Inspection Report	CG-5145	COMDTINST M6240.4 (series) Chap 11.	

Table 9-A-3

Reports Required Quarterly

Report Name	Format or Form Required	Reference	Frequency or Date
Controlled Substances Audit Board	Perpetual Inventory of Narcotics, Alcohol and Controlled Drugs, NAVMED 6710/5 and CG5353.	Chapter 10. Section B of this Manual	No later than 5th working day of the month following end of quarter.

Table 9-A-4

Reports Required "As Needed"

Report Name	Format or Form Required	Reference	Frequency or Date
Readiness Report	locally designed form	See Paragraph 2-(g) of this section.	Monthly (or as directed by command).
Injury Report for Not Misconduct and In-Line-of-Duty Determination	CG-3822	See Paragraph 8 of this Section	As needed. See Paragraph 8 of this Section.
Disease Alert Reports	RCN 6000-4	See chapter 7-B of this Manual	As needed
Inpatient Hospitalization Report	e-mail	See chapter 2-A. of this Manual	As needed
Report of Potential Third Party Liability	CG-4899	COMDTINST 6010.16 (series) and Chapter 11-B of this Manual	As needed
Potable Water Quality Discrepancy Report		COMDTINST M6240.5 (series)	when potable water quality fails to meet requirements or is suspect
Emergency Medical Treatment Report	CG 5214	COMDTINST M16135.4 (series)	As needed

7. <u>Combat Operations</u>.

   a. <u>Battle Dressing Station (BDS)</u>. The Health Services Allowance List contains a list of all items required in the BDS. Inspect BDS supplies monthly and inventory quarterly to ensure adequate and full inventory. Check sterile supplies and re-sterilize every six months. Replace expired or deteriorated supplies and materials. Enter an appropriate entry in the health services log indicating that the inspection was conducted and the action taken. Report significant discrepancies to the Command.

   b. <u>Route and Access Marking to the BDS</u>. On cutters that have a BDS, the routes to the BDS shall be marked in accordance with the Coatings and Color Manual, COMDTINST M10360.3 (series). In general:

      (1) Self adhering Red Cross decals in both photo-luminescene (internal) and nonphoto-luminescene (exterior marking) are authorized.

(2) When establishing and marking the routes to the various stations throughout the cutter, the markers shall be located frequently enough to enable the person following the route to have a clear view of the next marker of the route to be followed.

(a) On the interior surfaces of the cutter, the signs shall be placed not less than 12 inches above the deck and no higher than 36 inches above the deck.

(b) On exterior surfaces, signs shall be placed approximately 60 inches above the deck.

(c) Label plates with red letters will be installed at each direct access to BDS.

(d) An adhesive reflective marking system will be used and maintained. The purpose of this system is to provide emergency information during a situation involving the loss of lighting.

c. Use of BDS. On cutters with separate BDSs, the BDS is not to be used for any purpose other than the treatment of injured personnel in an emergency situation. No items are to be placed in a manner which will block access or restrict use of the BDS.

d. First Aid Kits, Gun Bags and Portable Medical Lockers. Supplies stored in emergency medical kits (first aid kits, gun bags, and portable medical lockers) must be protected from weather and pilferage, and will be maintained as directed in the Health Services Allowance List. An inventory list for each kit will be maintained and a monthly inspection of all first aid kits, gun bags and portable medical lockers will be performed by the IDHS. Each kit will be secured with a wire seal or other anti-pilferage device that will indicate when it has been accessed. Each kit will be inspected monthly for tampering (seal intact). The inspection will be noted in the Health Services Log. Once per quarter, the contents of all first aid kits, gun bags and portable medical lockers will be inventoried. The inspection will be noted in the Health Services Log. Report significant discrepancies to the Command.

e. Oxygen Cylinders. Ensure that oxygen handling and storage precautions are posted next to all oxygen cylinders onboard the vessel. Oxygen is considered a drug and under no circumstances will oxygen be used for any purpose other than patient care. Oxygen cylinders (for ready use) must have the content level read every morning by the HS in order to ensure readiness in case of an emergency. Empty cylinders will be clearly tagged as empty and stored separately from full cylinders. Oxygen cylinders must be hydrostatically tested every 5 years. Damage Control Department personnel will be a good source of information on where to have Oxygen cylinders refilled or hydrostatically tested. Oxygen for medical use must be grade D.

8. Environmental Health. Environmental health program related activities make up a large percentage of the daily responsibility of the IDHS. For the purposes of this chapter, environmental health encompasses the disciplines of preventive

medicine, sanitation and occupational health. An effective environmental health program requires the IDHS to have a working knowledge of a large number of unit systems and work processes. An aggressive program of inspection and observation is required. These include:

a. Environmental Health Inspection. The IDHS will make routine daily messing and berthing space "walk through inspections" and make note of any conditions that require immediate action. These "walk through inspections" should be done in an informal manner but items requiring correction will be brought to the attention of the department head responsible for the area in question. The following shall be inspected daily:

(1) Living spaces.

(2) Heads and washrooms.

(3) Fresh provisions received (particularly milk and ice cream).

(4) Scullery in operation.

(5) Drinking fountains.

(6) Garbage disposals.

(7) Sewage disposals.

(8) Coffee messes.

(9) Water supplies.

(10) Industrial activities. (See Chapter 7 of this Manual and the Food Service Sanitation Manual, COMDTINST 6240.4 (series))

b. Food Service Sanitation. The Food Service Sanitation Manual, COMDTINST M6240.4 (series) provides in-depth information regarding food service sanitation. This section is intended to provide information specific to the duties of an IDHS on an afloat unit. In general, the IDHS will monitor the food service operation to ensure the protection of the crew from food borne illnesses. The duties of the IDHS will include:

(1) Maintain sanitary oversight of the galley and all food service, preparation, storage and scullery spaces. Such oversight includes stores on-load, storage, preparation, and serving of food; disposal of garbage; proper cleaning and sanitizing of equipment and utensils; personal hygiene of food handlers; proper storage temperature of food products, and the condition and cleanliness of the spaces.

(2) Food service areas will be inspected weekly. Specifically including food handlers, refrigerators, chill boxes, galley spaces, and pantries. The findings will be reported on a Food Services Establishment Inspection Report, Form CG-5145 and an appropriate entry shall be made in the health services log.

(3) Conduct an inspection of the subsistence items and food for fitness for human consumption. Ensure that subsistence items were received from

sources approved by the U.S. Department of Agriculture (USDA) or an approved source from a foreign port that complies with all laws relating to food and food labeling.

    (4) Conduct an initial physical screening of food service personnel for detection of any condition or communicable disease that could result in transmission of disease or food borne illness.

c. Storage of Food Items. Proper storage procedures play a major role in preventing food borne illnesses. The IDHS will make routine inspections of food storage areas to ensure that spaces are properly maintained to prevent supplies from being:

    (1) Infested by insects and rodents.

    (2) Contaminated by sewage, chemicals, or dirt.

    (3) Subsistence items will be inspected by the HS upon receipt to determine food quality and ensure the stores are free from insect or rodent infestation. The results of this inspection will be recorded in the Health Services Log.

d. Coffee Mess. Food consumption, with the exception of coffee and condiments, will be limited to messing areas and lounges. Coffee messes provide a potential food source for insects and rodents if they are not properly located and kept scrupulously clean. For these reasons, permission to establish a coffee mess must be obtained from the Commanding Officer by the department desiring to establish a mess prior to its establishment. Messes will be physically located in a place that can be easily cleaned. Food contact areas (surrounding counter or table tops) must be non porous and kept free of spillage and food debris. Strict sanitary measures are to be used. Coffee mess regulations specifying sanitary operation of the mess will be posted. Use of community cups and spoons are prohibited. Inspection of coffee messes may be documented using a Food Service Sanitation Inspection Report, Form CG-5145 or through a locally generated inspection report form.

e. Water Supply. Water is used by all members of ship's company and so a tremendous potential exists for ship wide illness should potable water not be properly loaded from sources free from contamination, protected from contamination onboard, and a halogen residual maintained in the potable water tanks and throughout the distribution system. The IDHS will be notified whenever the potable water distribution system is opened for maintenance or repair. Establishment of a working relationship with the ship's Auxiliary Engineering Department and the "Fuel Oil Water King" will aid the IDHS in maintaining a proactive stance in regard to prevention of contamination of the vessel's potable water. The IDHS will make a monthly inspection of the potable water system and report conditions with potential to affect the health of the crew to the Commanding Officer.

(1) <u>Halogen Residual Testing</u>. Perform water tests for chlorine/bromine content daily outside of CONUS and at all units that make or chlorinate/brominate their own water and record the results in the Health Services Log. Consult the Water Supply and Wastewater Disposal Manual, COMDTINST M6240.5 (series).Chlorine/Bromine residual testing will also be performed before receiving any water onboard, and also 30 minutes after an initial halogenation has been accomplished. The Color Comparator Test set may be used for determining Halogen and pH levels. Nomenclature and ordering information is available in the HSAL. Four test sites should be selected: forward, aft, amidships and as far above the 0-1 deck as possible. This will give the widest range of sample points. Lack of a residual or a residual reading that is significantly lower than results at the other locations indicate possible contamination. Systematic testing from areas with low residuals "backward" to areas with "average" residuals will help locate the source or general area of contamination.

(2) <u>Bacteriological Test of Water</u>. Weekly, a potable water sample for bacteriological analysis will be collected from one of the four test sites selected for halogen residual testing. This includes a sample(s) collected directly from the potable water tanks and potable water retained in storage tanks when under direct service from shorelines. Samples of ice must also be collected from any machines making ice used for human consumption and tested for bacteriological growth. The results of bacteriological testing will be entered into the Potable Water Quality Log.

f. <u>Habitability</u>. The need for sanitary and hygienic living and working spaces is essential for good health and morale of the crew. General guidance on habitability standards can be found in the Safety and Environmental Health Manual COMDTINST M5100.47 (series), 5-D-1. Habitability inspection can most easily be accomplished if it is made a part of the material inspection of all ship's spaces normally scheduled by each command.

g. <u>Barber Shops</u>. Any space used for cutting hair may be designated a barber shop by the command. It will not be located in food service areas or berthing areas. Sanitation inspection of the ship's barber shop will be performed on a schedule determined by the command. General guidance on standards can be found in the, Safety and Environmental Health Manual, COMDTINST M5100.47 (series), 5-D-1-d-(6).

h. <u>Ship's Laundry</u>. Laundry spaces will be maintained in a clean and sanitary condition. Because of the potential for elevated temperature and high humidity within the space when laundry equipment is in operation, the ship's laundry will be identified as a heat stress monitoring space and monitored accordingly. Sanitation inspection of the ship's laundry will be performed on a schedule determined by the command. General guidance on standards can be found in the Safety and Environmental Health Manual COMDTINST M5100.47 (series), 5-D-1-d-(5).

i. <u>Fitness and Exercise Facilities</u>. The fitness and exercise facility will be inspected for cleanliness and compliance with general sanitation standards on a schedule determined by the command. General guidance on standards can be found in Chapter 2 of Manual of Naval Preventive Medicine, P-5010 (series).

j. <u>Insect Control</u>. Roaches, stored product pests, and to a lesser degree flies, can have significant impact on the health and general morale of a ship's company. Insect control starts in the warehouse from which stores are received. When practical, a visit by the IDHS to assess storage conditions can help decrease numbers of pests brought on board. Dockside inspection of all food stores brought on board is a must if insects are to be excluded. Produce with "loose" husks or skin such as onions provide common harborage for roaches as does the corrugation of cardboard boxes. Careful inspection with a good light and adjuncts such as an aerosolized flushing agent can identify harborages from which cans and stores can be removed prior to their being brought aboard. General guidance on standards can be found in the Safety and Environmental Health Manual COMDTINST M5100.47 (series), 5-D-3.

(1) <u>Roach Control</u>. A ship provides myriad harborages for roaches. Frequent and regular surveillance by the IDHS using a good light and a flushing agent can pinpoint areas of infestation. Roach traps containing pheromones work well in areas with small or isolated infestations. Larger or more widespread areas must be controlled initially with insecticide. Insecticide application will be made only by HSs that hold current certification to apply pesticides. Such personnel have been properly trained in pesticide selection, application, safety and handling precautions. This training is available through Navy Environmental Preventive Medicine Units (NEPMUs). Pesticide application may be available through Coast Guard Bases with attached Preventive Medicine Technicians. Any insect surveillance activity, general report of findings, or pesticide application, will be reported in the Health Services Log. Pest control services may also be contracted for from civilian pest control firms. Such services are paid for from ships AFC-30 funds and are contracted in the same manner as any other contract for services. While proper selection and application of the materials used is the legal responsibility of the licensed pest control operator, the IDHS must be informed of all applications made. The contractor must provide a report of pest control operations which includes, trade and chemical name of product used, strength and formulation applied, type of application (crack and crevice, etc), location of application. Requirement for such a report will be included in the contract for services. Report of pest control operations will be held on file for 3 years.

    (2) <u>Stored Products Pests</u>. A relatively small infestation of flour, grains, beans and cereals with stored products pests can spread quickly and lead to the loss of most or all of such products in a storage area if an infestation is not identified quickly and action taken to control it. In general, such action consists of identifying infested or suspect lots, removing them from storage with other food stuffs with the potential to become infested, and application of pesticide to control flying insects. Underway, control is limited to identification of infested or suspect lots and their removal.

    (3) <u>Rodent Control</u>.

        (a) Exclusion is by far the most effective means of rodent control available to the IDHS. Proper installation of rat guards is required on all mooring and service lines when the vessel is in port. Information about proper installation of rat guards can be found in Chapter 8 of the Manual of Naval Preventive Medicine, NAVMED P-5010 (series) and in the Safety and Environmental Health Manual, COMDTINST M5100.47 (series). The IDHS will inspect all mooring and service lines upon arrival in any port, including home port, to verify the proper placement of rat guards on all of the lines.

        (b) In the event that rodents do gain access to the vessel, an aggressive campaign using traps and/or poisoned bait (if the IDHS has been properly trained to apply and use such substances) must be undertaken. Trapping is the preferred method. Assistance may be available from Coast Guard Bases with attached Preventive Medicine Technicians or through the HSWL SC.

        (c) A current deraterization exemption certificate (Coast Guard Shipboard Sanitation Control Exemption Certificate/Ship Sanitation Control Certificate (SSCEC/SSCC), Form CG-5100B) must be kept onboard at all times. The certificate may be obtained from Coast Guard Bases with attached Preventive Medicine Technician; Navy units or bases with attached Preventive Medicine Technicians or NEPMUs. The deraterization certificate must be renewed every 6 months and must be included as a pre-deployment checklist item.

k. <u>Immunizations and Prophylaxis</u>. The IDHS will ensure that all personnel receive required immunizations in accordance with Immunizations and Chemoprophylaxis, COMDTINST 6230.4 (series). IDHS are only authorized to immunize active duty and reserve personnel. HSWL SC and NEPMUs can provide up to date information on immunization requirements, disease intelligence and preventive medicine precautions required for vessels deploying to OCONUS ports.

l. <u>Safety</u>. Dangers inherent to the shipboard environment are heightened by worker's lack of attention, short-cuts, "horseplay," inadequate training or understanding of a job or process, fatigue or over-familiarity. The IDHS must remain vigilant in regard to the safety and safe work practices of the crew. A safe work environment can't be maintained from the Health Services Department space. The IDHS must become familiar with the work processes that are on-going and be able to recognize when they are not being done in the proper manner or with the proper materials.

(1) Mishap Reporting. When accidents or mishaps do occur, certain reports or action may be required. The Safety and Environmental Health Manual, COMDTINST M5100.47 (series) contains requirements and guidance about mishap reporting. Such reports are not normally completed by the IDHS, but input may be required regarding severity of injury and required treatment.

(2) Accident Reports. The Administrative Investigations Manual, COMDTINST 5830.1 (series) contains a requirement that an Injury Report for Not Misconduct and In-Line-of-Duty Determination, Form CG-3822 be completed whenever an injury results in temporary or permanent disability. This report is referred to in the Physical Disability Evaluation System, COMDTINST M1850.2 (series) as a "Line of Duty (LOD) Report" and must be completed for all initial medical boards involving or resulting from trauma. Since it is difficult to determine the outcome of a serious injury in the early stages of treatment, an Injury Report For Not Misconduct and In Line of Duty Determination, Form CG-3822 (also commonly known as an "Accident Report") is usually completed in such cases. It is not necessary to complete an "Accident Report" for any and all injuries unless command policy dictates otherwise.

m. Vessel's Safety Board. The IDHS is a required member of the vessel's Safety Board. The IDHS should strive to be an active participant in the board, to identify potential problems or accident trends and suggest solutions to current or potential safety problems. Be proactive. Educate supervisors whenever possible.

n. Hazard Communication. The Hazard Communication Program is a unit wide program. Each unit will have appointed a Hazardous Materials Control Officer with overall responsibility for carrying out the program. Safety and Environmental Health Manual, COMDTINST M5100.47 (series) and Hazard Communication for Workplace Materials, COMDTINST 6260.21 (series) contain in-depth information about this program. The IDHS must be aware of the program requirements and its impact upon the operation of the Health Services Department. Additionally, the IDHS must know the location of the unit's central MSDS file and have immediate access to product information which may be needed to render proper treatment to exposed crewmembers. Computerized databases available on CD-ROM are acceptable for this purpose if the Health Services Department contains appropriate access to the information.

o. Heat Stress Program. Cutter Heat Stress Program, COMDTINST M6260.17 (series) provides details about this program. All areas of the vessel that expose crewmembers to extreme heat will have a dry bulb thermometer installed. Such areas normally include (but are not limited to) ship's laundry, scullery and engine room spaces. A Wet Bulb Globe Thermometer (WBGT) apparatus must be used to determine stay times of personnel working within heat hazardous spaces or areas and so familiarity with this equipment is required. The apparatus is normally operated by the IDHS or member of the engineering department. Recommendations for safe work rest cycles will be provided by the IDHS to the Engineering Watch Officer (EWO). Cutter Heat Stress Program, COMDTINST M6260.17 (series) provides information about the program. The WBGT is listed on the Health Services Allowance List (HSAL) and is procured as health care equipment. A Coast Guard Health Care Equipment Request, Form CG-5211 should be submitted to the HSWL SC. Current calibration of the ship's WBGT apparatus is a Tailored Annual Cutter Training "critical" item. Delinquent calibration can result in cancellation of some or all TACT drills by the training evaluation team. Contact the HSWL SC for locations to send WBGTs for calibration.

p. Sight Conservation Program. Eye protection and safety should be stressed in the workplace. Safety glasses or goggles will be provided for all crewmembers involved in eye-hazardous tasks. Tools with strong potential for eye hazard will be identified with an adhesive warning label. Fixed machinery with eye hazard potential will have posted nearby an easily visible warning placard, and eye protection will be easily accessible and clearly visible.

q. Eyewash Stations. Eyewash stations will be located in any space or work area with strong potential for splashes to, or foreign body injury of the eye. Eyewash stations will be maintained in accordance with the station's manufacturer requirements. Eyewash stations shall be flushed weekly for 15 seconds and flushed and drained according to the recommendations of the biostat ingredient manufacturer used in the station. This interval is usually every six months. Eyewash stations will be "tagged" with a maintenance record tag and inspection or maintenance activities will be recorded when performed. Inspections of eyewash stations will be recorded in the Health Services Log.

B. **Independent Duty Ashore at Sectors, Sector Field Offices, Air Stations, and Small Boat Stations.**

1. **Introduction.** The identification or term Independent Duty Health Services Technician, used in any form, only identifies those Health Services Technicians that have successfully completed one of the three recognized Independent Duty Training courses, i.e. the USCG Independent Duty Health Services Technician, USN Independent Duty Corpsman, or USAF Independent Duty Medical Technician courses. Assignment to independent duty is challenging. The role is one of tremendous responsibility and at times can tax even the most experienced HS's skill, knowledge and ability. Along with the increased responsibility and sometimes arduous duty comes the potential for personal satisfaction unsurpassed by any other job assignment. An Independent Duty Health Services (IDHS) Ashore is a Health Services Technician assigned to an ashore unit such as a Sector, Sector Field Office, Air Station, or Small Boat Station without an MO attached.

2. **Mission, General Duties and Responsibilities.**

   a. **Mission.** The Health Services Technician serving at an ashore unit is charged with the responsibility for the prevention and control of disease and injury, and the treatment of the sick and injured. It is recognized that IDHSs assigned to an ashore unit are responsible for ensuring personnel assigned to units within their parent command's area of responsibility (AOR) maintain their fitness for duty and medical readiness. This oversight requires the IDHS to work closely with unit Executive Officers (XO)/Executive Petty Officers (XPO) to ensure unit personnel are up to date on medical readiness items such as, immunizations, required lab tests, physical and dental exams and are receiving the necessary medical training in order to perform their jobs.

   b. **General Duties.** HSs on independent duty perform the administrative duties and, to the extent for which qualified clinical duties (See United States Coast Guard Regulations 1992, COMDTINST M5000.3 (series)). They shall not attempt, nor be required to provide, health care for which they are not professionally qualified. They shall provide care only for AD personnel; however, they may provide care to non-active duty patients on an emergency basis. The filling of prescriptions for other than AD personnel shall be strictly limited to emergency situations and to authorized stock on hand under the allowance list for the unit. They may, under the guidance set in Chapter 10 of this Manual, establish non-prescription medication programs for eligible beneficiaries.

   c. **Responsibilities.** The Commanding Officer (CO) is responsible for the health and readiness of the command. The health services department is charged with advising the CO of conditions existing that may be detrimental to the health of personnel and for making appropriate recommendations for correcting such conditions. Meticulous attention to all details and aspects of preventing disease must be a continuing program. It is imperative that unit sanitation and preventive health practices be reviewed constantly in order that any disease promoting situation may be discovered immediately and promptly eradicated. In the absence of a permanently attached MO the CO will designate a member (generally the Executive Officer (XO) or Logistics Officer (LOGO)) to have direct responsibility for medical matters. The role of the IDHS is to assist the command in maintaining the good health and physical readiness of the crew. To accomplish this, the IDHS must be informed of planned operations and anticipate any operational demands resulting from such operations. To this end, the IDHS will consult and advise the command in all matters with potential to effect crew readiness or the health of personnel. Some of the duties of the IDHS include but are not limited to:

(1) Assessment and treatment of illness and injury. Hold daily sick call if applicable. Diagnose and treat patients within capabilities. When indicated, refer cases to facilities where Medical or Dental Officers are available or, if this is not practical, obtain help and advice by radio or other expeditious means.

(2) Prevention of illness and injury through an aggressive environmental health program. Such a program includes inspection of living and working spaces, food service and storage areas, and food storage and handling practices, integrated pest management practices, potable water quality surveillance, and recognition and management of communicable diseases.

(3) Provision of Health Services training aligned with the needs and mission of the unit.

(4) Security and proper use of health services supplies, material and property.

(5) Maintenance and documentation of medical and dental readiness of personnel within their unit's AOR. The IDHS will assist the command in ensuring the medical and dental readiness for the personnel in their AOR by providing monthly CGBI Medical and Dental Readiness, scheduling the crew for required readiness exams and procedures as needed, and informing the command when a given crew member or command fails to cooperate with the IDHS's efforts to comply with readiness requirements. The IDHS shall also maintain a tickler system to include all return appointments requested by physicians or dentists from outside referrals requested by the command.

(6) Supply and logistics to ensure supplies, materials and equipment necessary to carry out the mission of the Health Services Department are obtained and maintained in sufficient quantity and condition to support the unit mission and operation.

(7) Health Services Department administration, maintenance, and security of health records. Maintain health records as required by Chapter 4 of this Manual. Ensure that all treatment records and/or consults from outside referrals are obtained and placed in the health record. In addition, ensure that each patient is notified of all physical exams, consultations, and diagnostic tests (e.g., pap smears, mammograms, biopsies, x-rays, etc.) performed at any facility prior to filing in the health record. Maintain the security and

confidentiality of all medical/dental records, databases and any other protected health information

(8) Strict adherence to Chapter 2 of this Manual which contains information about general and specific duties of the HS serving independently, including all required training in compliance with HIPAA privacy and security.

(9) Other duties as assigned by the CO. In accordance with Paragraph 7-5-4, United States Coast Guard Regulations 1992, COMDTINST M5000.3 (series), HS may not be detailed to perform combatant duties in their own defense or protection of the wounded and sick in their charge, which are not prohibited by the Geneva Conventions. However, under routine situations; HSs who bear arms forfeit the special protections for medical personnel afforded by the Geneva Convention.

3. Chain Of Command. The IDHS will report directly to the Executive Officer (XO) or Logistics Officer as dictated by the CO.

4. Operation of the Health Services Division. The IDHS Ashore Health Services Division is classified as a 1-D (ashore) sickbay. The unit may request a waiver from maintaining the full allowance list. This request will be routed to the assigned Designated Medical Officer advisor (DMOA), SIDHS and HSWL SC for approval. The IDHS is tasked with a wide variety and high volume of duties and responsibilities. This section sets forth policy and guidelines designed to assist the IDHS in carrying out assigned duties and responsibilities.

a. Health Services Division Standard Operating Procedure. In order to successfully manage the Health Services Division, the IDHS must use time management and organizational skills and tools. One such tool is a written Standard Operating Procedure (SOP) for the Health Services Division. The SOP will govern the activities of the IDHS, and has as its guiding precept, the goals and missions of the unit. The SOP will be developed and submitted in written form to the CO for approval via the chain of command. In addition, the SOP will be reviewed, updated to reflect current policies and procedures and signed at least annually by the IDHS, DMOA, XO and CO. The approved SOP will be kept in the Health Services Division for easy referral. Copies of pertinent sections will be posted as appropriate. The SOP will include:

(1) A copy of the IDHS's letter of assumption of duties as Health Services Division Representative.

(2) A copy of the IDHS's prescribing formulary approved by the DMOA.

(3) A written daily schedule of events for both on base and deployed periods.

(4) Copies of all letters of designation, assignment, and authority that directly impact upon the IDHS or Health Services Division. Examples include those granting "By direction" authority, designation as working Narcotics and Controlled Substances custodian, written certification to provide immunizations (see Chapter 7 Section C) and assignment of a DMOA.

(5) A copy of the unit's organizational structure. This document will show graphically the IDHS's chain of command.

(6) A listing of duties and responsibilities assigned to the IDHS and the frequency that they are to be carried out. The listing will include both primary and collateral assigned duties.

(7) A listing of all required reports, the format required for submission, the frequency or date required, required routing and required "copy addressees". Incorporation of this information in tabular format provides a quick and easy guide for reference purposes.

(8) Guidance on how any change in a member's duty status is relayed from the member through the IDHS to the XO or Logistics Officer as dictated by the CO.

(9) A unit instruction or SOP for the management of rape or sexual assault cases. The document must provide policy for the Health Services Department action in such cases, names of organizations, points of contact and telephone numbers for local resources as well as contact information for agencies and facilities which must be notified. CGIS must be notified for all unrestricted reports of alleged rape or sexual assault. It must contain a prearranged mechanism for timely completion of a physical examination by a **SAMFE or SANE** for the purpose of evidence gathering that meets requirements of all applicable law enforcement agencies. Additionally, it must define limitations that will exist if the unit is underway at the time the incident occurs. It must contain directions on how to complete a Victim Reporting Preference Statement, Form CG-6095. **Additionally, it must define the unrestricted and restricted reporting procedures as outlined in the Sexual Assault Prevention and Response (SAPR) Program, COMDTINST M1754.10 (series).**

(10) A unit instruction or SOP section for the management of suicide threat or attempt. The document must provide policy for Health Services Division action in such cases, names of organizations, points of contact and telephone numbers for local resources, contact information for agencies and facilities which must be notified as well as a listing of required information, reports or actions.

(11) A unit instruction or SOP section for the management of family violence. The document must provide policy for Health Services Division action in such cases, names of organizations, points of contact and telephone numbers for local resources, contact information for agencies and facilities which must be notified as well as a listing of required information, reports or actions.

b. Departure from the Daily Schedule of Events. The day-to-day operation of the Health Services Department is complex and has the potential to be impacted by the operational needs of the unit. It will, of necessity, change when events of higher priority or concern occur. When deviation from the daily schedule of events is required, notifying the chain of command will occur at the earliest opportunity. When deviation from the daily schedule of events occurs frequently, the daily schedule of events will be reviewed and if necessary, changed. Any changes will be incorporated into the Health Services Division SOP and approved by the Commanding Officer.

c. Relief and Assumption of Duties as the IDHS. Proper documentation of the status of the Health Services Division and the condition of its equipment, stores, and records is required at the time of relief and assumption of the duties and responsibilities as the IDHS. This must be completed in order to adequately ascertain the state of operational medical readiness of the health services department and advise the local command. Operational readiness refers to the immediate ability to meet all health care demands within the unit's capabilities. The process is complex and requires both the incoming and outgoing IDHS to jointly perform the following:

(1) A complete inventory of all medical stores, spaces, and equipment, including durable medical equipment. Obtain the unit Health Services Allowance List and inspect the inventory of all health services department equipment, supplies, and publications. Initiate action for repair, survey, or replenishment of equipment, supplies, and publications. Verify inventory records and check all logs. Report any discrepancies to the local command without delay. Amplification of requirements and procedures is contained in Chapters 8 and 10 of this Manual. Health Services Allowance List, Ashore COMDTINST M6700.5 (series) provides a listing of supplies and the equipment required.

(a) A controlled substances inventory must be done. Use direction provided in Chapter 10 of this Manual.

(b) A complete inventory of all unit property in custody of the Health Services Division if the IDHS is the custodian of the property shall be completed.

(2) A review of ongoing actions affecting the status of the Health Services Division such as, outstanding requisitions, survey or repairs, and proper documentation of all such transactions.

(3) A review of the Health Services Division SOP.

(4) A review of the most recent HSWL SC Quality Improvement Survey for the unit. A copy of the survey annotated with any finding of incomplete or uncorrected discrepancies will be included as an enclosure to the letter of relief.

(5) Check health records against the personnel roster. Any missing records should be accounted for or requested from previous duty stations. If records cannot be accounted for within one month's time, open a new health record. Check health records for completeness, and if not current, obtain and enter

all missing information to the fullest extent possible. (See Chapter 4 of this Manual for further instructions pertaining to health records).

d. <u>Letter of Relief and Assumption of Duties</u>. Upon completion of the Health Services Division review, a memorandum will be prepared and submitted by the incoming IDHS via the chain of command and will advise the Commanding Officer of the status of the Health Services Division. A copy of the letter will be forwarded to the HSWL SC Senior IDHS Team Leader. The letter of Relief and Assumption of Duties will provide the following:

(1) Date of assumption of duties; a statement that the duties and responsibilities of the IDHS have been assumed; and a thorough review of the Health Services Division has been conducted. Any discrepancies of material or record keeping will be annotated on a copy of the unit's most recent HSWL SC Quality Improvement Survey and submitted as an enclosure to the letter of Relief and Assumption of Duties as IDHS.

(2) Any discrepancies noted upon relief will be handled as a matter of individual command prerogative. Responsibility for correction, adjustment of account or inventory records, action required to replace missing items, as well as any necessary disciplinary action will be determined by the command.

(3) In cases in which no on site relief occurs, all of the preceding action will be completed. The supply officer of the unit will participate in the review process in place of the outgoing IDHS.

e. <u>Actions upon Proper Relief</u>. Upon assumption of duties as the unit's IDHS, one of the first tasks to complete is a thorough review of all SOPs and department instructions. A check of the references should be accomplished in order to ensure established point of contacts for the local area are verified and updated as needed. If possible, make visits and introductions in person. The IDHS must find out how each system works and how it is accessed.

5. <u>Providing Health Care</u>. Delivery of health care is undoubtedly the most challenging and rewarding part of the job of any IDHS. The IDHS assigned to an ashore unit will face the challenges of determining when to deliver care to patients and when it is necessary to refer patients to a higher level of care at a local health care facility (military or civilian). At times, the IDHS will be called upon to assist his/her command or a unit in his/her command's AOR in determining a member's fitness for duty. This section is intended to provide a brief summary of the various facets of providing this medical care.

a. <u>Medical Officer Advisor (DMOA)</u>. Each IDHS ashore shall be assigned a DMOA in accordance with Chapter 1 of this Manual. Good communication between the IDHS and DMOA can prevent many problems affecting health care delivery to personnel. The IDHS shall schedule a visit to the DMOA as soon as is practical after reporting to their unit or upon completion of IDHS School. The purpose of the visit is to allow first-hand communication between the DMOA and IDHS on expectations, support facility requirements, and any unique needs or concerns. This visit will normally be scheduled for a period of at least two weeks. This time frame will allow for the DMOA to evaluate the IDHS's performance factors and qualifications, and to develop a formulary for the IDHS. Open communication should be maintained through regular site visits when practical, or at minimum, regular telephone calls. With regard to provision of direct care, the IDHS will seek the DMOA's or another Medical Officer's (MO) advice whenever there are questions about a patient's condition or when the following conditions exist:

  (1) Return to sick call before assigned follow-up because of failure to improve or condition has deteriorated.

  (2) Member cannot return to full duty status after 72 hours duration because of unresolved illness or injury.

b. The IDHS should contact his/her DMOA when any of the following emergency conditions exist.

  (1) Fever of unknown origin of 102 degrees Fahrenheit or higher (when taken orally) persisting for 48 hours.

  (2) Fever of 103 degrees Fahrenheit or higher (when taken orally).

  (3) Unexplained pulse rate above 120 beats per minute.

  (4) Unexplained respiratory rate above 28 breaths per minute or less than 12 breaths per minute.

  (5) Psychosis or Depression with suicidal thoughts.

  (6) Change in mental status or level of consciousness.

  (7) Chest pain or arrhythmia.

  (8) Unexplained shortness of breath.

  (9) Rape or sexual assault.

  (10) Any condition threatening life or limb.

c. Gender Considerations. Chapter 1.Section B of this Manual provides specific direction for health services technicians about patient privacy, same gender attendant requirements, and examination restrictions.

d. Avoiding Common Problems. Scheduling and obtaining the routine medical care required by personnel can tax the organizational skills of even the most experienced IDHS. There are, however, actions that the IDHS can take which will enhance the chances of getting the routine appointments needed for all members. Some of these are:

  (1) Identify the routine medical and dental needs of unit personnel. The IDHS's supporting Coast Guard (CG) clinic, Department of Defense Medical Treatment Facility (DoD MTF) or civilian primary care manager have established appointment scheduling procedures which the IDHS must work within whenever time allows. Follow the requirements for

scheduling all appointments. When routine medical or dental care is to be made directly to a DoD MTF, the IDHS must determine the facility's requirements for referral of patients and follow any local procedures.

(2) Communicate with the supporting clinic often. Discuss the unit's medical and dental needs with the clinic supervisor and DMOA (if located at the facility).

(3) Perform all preliminary tests and complete all necessary paperwork before scheduling physical exams at the supporting clinic.

(4) Post a listing of appointment dates and times as soon as they become available. Provide each Department/Division Chief with a listing of the appointments applicable to their division or shop.

(5) Hold members accountable for being at their appointed place and time. Provide feedback to division officers and shop chiefs on appointment failures. Notify the XO or XPO if members fail to show for more than one appointment.

e. Consultations. During the management of complex or protracted cases, consultations or specialty referral may be necessary. When such services are needed, the IDHS will normally make referral to a CG clinic, or in some cases, a DoD MTF. When referring a patient to see a Medical Officer at a CG clinic, the IDHS shall ensure that a Chronological Record of Care, Form SF-600 entry is completed using the SOAP format and that an appointment is scheduled. The clinic will normally provide treatment or arrange care if treatment is beyond its scope. When consultations or referral for specialty care are made directly to a DoD MTF, the IDHS must determine the facility requirements for referral of patients and follow any local procedures. Referrals to a DoD MTF will normally be documented using a Consultation Sheet, Form SF-513 or a Referral for Civilian Medical Care, Form DD-2161. The consultation will provide a concise history of the condition to be evaluated as well as any pertinent findings. A provisional diagnosis is normally expected by the consultant. Chapter 4 Section B. of this Manual provides direction on completion of a Consultation Sheet, Form SF-513. The patient and the patient's supervisor must be informed of all consultation or referral appointment dates and times. Professional courtesy is an important part of maintaining good working relationships with the facilities that the IDHS accesses for consultation and referral. Timely notification to the referral facility when appointment changes or cancellations occur (along with a brief explanation of why the change is required) helps maintain those relationships. Whenever possible, provide at least 24 hours notice for changes or cancellations.

f. Antibiotic Therapy. The IDHS may prescribe and administer antibiotics included on the Health Services Allowance List. Whenever possible, the IDHS shall consult with their DMOA or other Medical Officer for a recommendation or concurrence prior to administering antibiotic therapy.

g. Health Services Division Treatment Space. The Health Services Division treatment space will be manned at all times when patients are inside. All items are to be stowed in their proper place and secured. All medical records shall be locked in a cabinet. At no time should the Health Services space be left unlocked when the IDHS is not in the space.

h. Convalescent Leave/Sick Leave. Convalescent leave/Sick leave is a period of leave not charged against a member's leave account. It can be a recommendation to the command when a patient is Not Fit For Duty (usually for a duration expected to be greater than 72 hours) and whose recovery time can reasonably be expected to improve by freedom from the confines of quarters. It should be considered only when required as an adjunct to patient treatment. The command must evaluate each recommendation. Commands are authorized to grant convalescent leave as outlined in Military Assignments and Authorized Absences, M1000.8 (series).

i. Dental. The IDHS is responsible for arranging for the necessary dental examinations of unit personnel. All personnel must receive an annual dental exam and the results must be documented in DENCAS. See Chapter 2 of this Manual for guidance on obtaining dental services from contract dental providers.

j. Rape or Sexual Assault. **All victims of rape or sexual assault must be treated in a professional, compassionate and non-judgmental manner. The unit shall have an SOP for dealing with reported cases of alleged rape and sexual assault. Refer to the Sexual Assault prevention and Response (SAPR) Program, COMDTINST M1754.10 (series) for further guidance.**

k. Suicide Prevention. An encounter with a suicidal person is always a deeply emotional event. It is important for the IDHS to act in a caring and professional manner. Early intervention and good communication skills are essential. If suicidal ideation is suspected it is important to remember:

   (1) Take all threats and symptoms seriously. Immediately seek professional help from the nearest MTF or local health care facility for any member considering suicide. At no time should the person be left unattended. Once the patient is safe, contact the servicing Work-Life office for additional help or refer to Suicide Prevention Program, COMDTINST 1734.1 (series).

   (2) Actively listen to the patient. Do not argue, judge, attempt to diagnose, or analyze the person's true intentions. It is important to provide a calm, caring, professional demeanor throughout the entire situation. Thoroughly document the patient encounter using the SOAP format.

   (3) Arrange for an escort and a driver to transport the patient to the nearest CG clinic, DoD MTF or civilian emergency room with facilities appropriate to the situation. The unit's SOP for suicide threat or attempt should contain this information for ready use if needed.

l. Decedent Affairs. Chapter 5 of this Manual contains guidance about action that the Health Services Division must take when there is a death of a CG member. Military Casualties and Decedent Affairs, COMDTINST M1770.9 (series) contains further guidance concerning casualties and decedent affairs. It is unlikely that the IDHS will be assigned as the Casualty Assistance Calls Officer (CACO) for the command, but the IDHS will undoubtedly be heavily involved with the process of proper disposition of remains, so familiarity with the information required is helpful. The IDHS should also perform the following:

(1) Make an entry in the Health Services Log will be made detailing all available information concerning the death.

(2) Terminate the deceased member's health record in accordance with Chapter 4 of this Manual.

m. Disposition of Remains. As soon as possible, remains will be transferred to the nearest Military Treatment Facility (MTF) for further disposition. When transfer cannot be accomplished immediately, the remains will be placed into a body pouch and refrigerated at a temperature of 36 to 40 degrees Fahrenheit to prevent decomposition. The space must contain no other items and must be cleaned and disinfected before reuse. Remains will be identified with a waterproof tag, marked with waterproof ink, and affixed with wire ties to the right great toe of the decedent and also to each end of the body pouch. The minimum information needed on each tag includes the full name, SSN and rate or rank of the decedent. Whenever possible, do not remove items attached to the deceased at time of death. Such items may include (for example) IV lines, needles, AED pads, ET tubes, lengths of cord or line, etc. These may be important during an autopsy. Additionally, do not discard or launder clothing of the deceased. These items are sometimes important to surviving family members and in some cultures is part of the mourning process for the deceased. This is a cultural consideration but should be a part of the decision process.

n. Physical Disability Evaluation System. The medical board process is detailed in Military Separations, COMDTINST M1000.4 (series) and the Physical Disability Evaluation System, COMDTINST M1850.2 (series).

6. Training. The purpose of training for both the assigned IDHS and that provided to the unit includes: assurance that the IDHS and crewmembers are able to provide aid for themselves and their shipmates in an emergency situation and to promote the general health and well being of the unit.

a. Training for the IDHS. In addition to the requirements of the rate, the ashore IDHS must complete certain "C" schools. These are:

(1) CG Independent Duty Health Services Technician, Air Force Medical Services Craftsman or Navy Surface Forces Independent Duty Technician.

(2) CG Introduction to Environmental Health or Navy Basic Shipboard Series. (Note: This is not required for graduates of Navy Surface Forces Independent Duty Technician or Independent Duty Health Services Technician School).

(3) Emergency Medical Technician. IDHS are required to maintain currency with the National Registry of Emergency Medical Technicians (NREMT). Short Term Training Requests are to be completed in accordance with the Training and Education Manual, COMDTINST M1500.10 (series) and forwarded to Commandant (CG-1121). Funding will be provided by Commandant (CG-11). See the Emergency Medical Services Manual, COMDTINST M16135.4 (series) for additional information.

(4) Instructor courses (Must maintain current certification in) CPR, BLS, AED and First Responder.

(5) Field Management of Chemical and Biological Casualties. The Field Management of Chemical and Biological Casualties Course (FCBC) is conducted by the US Army Medical Research Institute of Chemical Defense (USAMRICD) at Aberdeen Proving Ground, Maryland. Classroom instruction, laboratory and field exercises prepare graduates to become trainers in the first echelon management of chemical and biological agent casualties.

b. IDHS Initial Certification. All newly assigned IDHSs will participate in an orientation and certification program at their supporting clinic. Initial orientation must be completed within 60 days of reporting in to the new unit. If due to operational commitments the orientation and certification can not be completed within 60 days of reporting, a waiver request must be sent in memo format to the HSWLSC, SIDHS Team Leader. If the unit is unable to fund the tdy, the IDHS shall request funding from their HSWL SIDHS. Initial orientation and certification is estimated to take 2 weeks. During this time, the IDHS will:

(1) Work with his/her DMOA to complete the IDHS Operational Integration Form, CG-6000-4.

(2) See a minimum of 12 patients

(3) Perform a focused exam on each of the body's systems while using the DMOA as a guide and evaluator.

(4) Discuss with his/her DMOA notification procedures for the dispensing of scheduled drugs, administration of emergency medications and antibiotics.

(5) Solicit documented feedback from the DMOA and work to improve any areas where required.

(6) Perform a minimum of 4 clinical hours with a dental preceptor.

(7) Solicit documented feedback from the dental preceptor and work to improve any areas where required.

(8) Demonstrate a verbal understanding of management of acute dental problems to include dental abscess, periodontal disease, temporary fillings, fractured teeth, etc.

(9) Demonstrate documentation requirements for dental problems.

   c. <u>IDHS Annual Sustainment Training Requirements</u>. Every 12 months, the IDHS must complete the following task:

     (1) <u>See a minimum of 48 patients/year</u>. The IDHS shall solicit feedback from his/her DMOA on the patients treated over the last year.

     (2) Work with his/her DMOA to complete the IDHS Operational Integration Form, CG-6000-4.

     (3) Instruct at least one BLS certification class.

     (4) Review all CEUs acquired over the last year in order to maintain EMT certification with his/her DMOA.

   d. <u>Health Services Department Training Plan</u>. A plan for training of unit personnel will be established in written form and kept on file. It will be based on a minimum 12 month cycle and be included in the unit training schedule. At a minimum, the following training will be given:

     (1) Basic first aid (to include shock, hemorrhage control, dressing, airway management and assisted ventilation and the use of items in first aid kits).

     (2) Personal and dental hygiene.

     (3) STI/HIV prevention.

     (4) Heat and cold stress programs, including hypothermia.

     (5) Respiratory protection program.

     (6) Hearing conservation.

     (7) Sight conservation.

     (8) Blood borne pathogens.

   e. <u>Documentation of Training</u>. Documentation of the training is a requirement. An outline must be prepared and kept on file for all training topics presented and a training log maintained for all training provided. The training log will contain a record of all HS training given to unit personnel. It will contain the following information:

     (1) Date.

     (2) Topic.

     (3) Duration.

     (4) Instructor's name.

     (5) Names and signatures of members attending training.

   f. <u>Training Format</u>. Training will normally be presented in either lecture format or demonstration and practical application. Lecture format presentations should be limited to 15 to 20 minutes and demonstrations and practical application should not exceed 1 hour. Practical application must be of high priority in training unit personnel in first aid, casualty evaluation, and treatment. There is no substitute for "hands on" practice in developing effective first aid skills.

7. Supply And Logistics.

a. Custody of Health Services Equipment and Material. As directed by the Commanding Officer, the IDHS is responsible and accountable for the health services material onboard the unit. As such, the IDHS is the custodian of all health service equipment and material. The custodian will not permit waste or abuse of supplies or equipment and will use techniques such as stock rotation, planned replacement and preventive maintenance to minimize waste of resources.

b. Inventory. An accurate record of medical stores and equipment must be maintained. The inventory of medical stores, spaces and equipment will be prepared using the Stock Record Card Afloat, NAVSUP-1114 or in line item form (computerized database is an approved and preferred alternative if all necessary information is captured) and include:

(1) Quantity and shelf-life of each item currently on board.

(2) Balance on hand, high-level, low-level (reorder point for each item).

(3) Manufacturer, lot number and expiration date (pharmaceuticals).

(4) Quantity placed on order, date received.

c. Unit Property. Unit property in Health Services Department custody must also be safeguarded and accounted for. The unit property custodian should be contacted before transfer or destruction of such property.

d. Funding and Account Record Keeping. Funds used to purchase supplies and equipment, and to pay for the various expenses of operating the unit are broken down into Allotment Fund Control code (AFC) expenditure categories. This method allows for efficient budgeting and accounting. Fund categories generally used by IDHSs fall within the AFC subhead 30 or 57 expenditure categories.

(1) AFC-30 is a general unit fund used by the supply department to purchase generally needed operating supplies and services. Examples include pens, paper, books, training aids, etc. AFC-30 funding can be used to pay for Health Services Department supplies and equipment not obtainable through Defense Supply Center Philadelphia Prime Vendor Program (via the unit's supporting clinic) or the major medical equipment request process (see Chapters 6 and 8 of this Manual). Restrictions exist on what may be purchased with AFC-30 funds. Unit supply personnel can answer specific questions.

(2) AFC-57 is a funding category used to purchase health care related supplies and equipment, and to pay for health care. AFC-57 funds are distributed to the HSWL SC and further allocated by them to the units within their areas of responsibility with IDHSs assigned.

(3) With the full implementation of the Prime Vendor programs for Pharmaceuticals and for Medical and Surgical Supplies, AFC-57 fund allocations will be made to the Prime Vendor ordering point assigned for the unit.

e. <u>Budgets and Budgeting</u>. In general, IDHSs do not need to plan and submit an AFC-57 budget request because medical supplies and equipment funding are controlled by the HSWL SC and Prime Vendor ordering points. If additional AFC-57 resource needs are anticipated, the IDHS's supporting clinic should be contacted for direction on how the resources are to be requested. The budget build process does have value for the IDHS however. AFC-30 funds will need to be planned for and requested from your unit. Medical equipment in need of replacement costing less than $500.00 must be requested from the supporting clinic. Medical equipment in need of replacement costing $500.00 or more must be requested from the HSWL SC via a Health Care Equipment Request, Form CG-5211. The budget build process is a good way to handle these needs. AFC-30 fund budget planning is relatively straight forward, although it can be time consuming. AFC-30 expenditures for Health Services should be broken into general use categories. Examples of categories are books and publications, non-consumable goods and services such as hydro testing and replacement of oxygen cylinders and annual calibration of heat stress meters, and travel for continuing education. Budgeting categories can be as simple or complicated as the IDHS desires to make it. Once categories have been established, a ledger for the Health Services Division should be "opened" and the expenditure categories entered into it. The use of a "spreadsheet" program is an efficient way to keep an accounting record, but a ledger book works just as well. Attention to detail is the key. In general, a system using four to five categories works well.

(1) In preparing a budget for the upcoming year, it is important to look back over what was purchased in the previous year. To do this, collect all records of AFC-30 orders and expenditures. Review each line item and record the amount spent into the appropriate budget category. The steps for preparing a budget and carrying it out along with general timelines are contained in this paragraph. They are:

Table 9-B-1

March	Look back process. Review amount of funds spent over the first two quarters of the fiscal year as well as spending patterns for the previous fiscal year. Note general categories on which funds were spent and in which quarter items were ordered. This will allow projection of quarterly funding needs into the upcoming year.
April/May	Review status of the Health Services Division medical library and determine which texts and references must be updated.
	Review status of HS certifications and continuing medical education. Funding for training, conferences or seminars not normally funded by AFC-56 funds must be budgeted for as AFC 30 budget line items.
	Review preventive maintenance records and include cost projections in AFC-30 budget. Prepare and submit U.S. Coast Guard Health Care Equipment Request, Form CG 5211s for medical equipment to be replaced.
	Seek guidance from XO on known or planned activities outside normal operations.
June	Submit finalized budget proposal through chain of command. AFC 30 budget information will be added to the unit budget. Be prepared to "defend" the budget request submitted. Documentation of the data gathering process and retrieval of the raw data used to justify the funding requested will likely be required. AFC-56 funds requests will be consolidated by the command and forwarded to the unit's district, HSWL SC or Area commander, as appropriate.

(2) Careful stewardship, good record keeping and accounting make existing funding and justification for increased funding levels easier.

f. Obtaining Pharmaceuticals, Medical and Surgical Supplies. Chapter 8 of this Manual provides policy applicable to the management of Health Services supplies. Prime Vendor programs for both Pharmaceuticals and Medical/Surgical Supplies have been established and it is through these programs that essentially all pharmaceuticals and supplies will be obtained. From an IDHS's perspective important aspects of the program include:

(1) Each unit has been assigned a Prime Vendor ordering point for Pharmaceuticals and for Medical/Surgical Supplies. The HSWL SC assigns the POCs and periodically updates the information. The Prime Vendor ordering point may be different for each of the programs.

(2) Funding for both Prime Vendor for Pharmaceuticals and Prime Vendor for Medical/Surgical Supplies is provided to the assigned Prime Vendor ordering point by the HSWL SC. Internal accounting procedures vary among Prime Vendor ordering points. Some have established individual accounts for the units they are responsible for while others manage funds from a central account. Regardless of the accounting method used by the Prime Vendor ordering point, the IDHS must establish and maintain a system to track expenditures.

(3) Prime Vendor ordering points establish pharmaceutical and medical/surgical supply ordering procedures for their assigned units. Pharmaceutical and medical supply items ordered will be those required by the Health Services Allowance List (HSAL) in quantities required for the unit type. Deviation from the HSAL requirements will normally occur only after justification of the need is made by the IDHS to the DMOA for the unit. It will be made in writing and kept on file for review during HSWL SC site surveys.

g. Health Services Supporting Clinic. The supporting clinic is the IDHS's partner in providing health care for the crew. Local agreements and resources may be available to allow the supporting clinic to provide a broader range of services to the IDHS and the crew but at a minimum, the following will be provided.

(1) All supplies and equipment (under $500.00) listed in the HSAL for the type of unit and on the HS Core Formulary. The unit no longer receives AFC-57 funding for the operation of the Health Services Division. These funds are provided instead to the supporting clinic with the intent that the supporting clinic will provide all required items for the IDHS to operate the Health Services Division.

(2) Assign the IDHS a DMOA in writing. The DMOA shall be available for questions about patient care, as well as completing record reviews quarterly.

(3) Perform medical boards for the IDHS unit as necessary.

(4) Provide a resource for advice and support in all administrative areas of health care delivery to include medical administration, physical examination review (within the approving authority of the Clinic Administrator), health benefits, medical billing and bill payment processing assistance, dental care, pharmacy administration, supply and logistics, bio-medical waste management, IDHS continuing education, and quality assurance support. Any services provided at the clinic shall be extended to the IDHS to the maximum extent possible.

h. <u>Preventive Maintenance of Health Services Equipment</u>. Chapter 8 Section D of this Manual details the preventive maintenance program for Health Services equipment. An important part of medical equipment readiness is a program of preventive maintenance and planned equipment replacement. Repair and routine replacement part costs should be recorded on a locally generated form or on side B of a Medical/Dental Equipment Maintenance Record, Form NAVMED 6700-3CG. Capture of this data will allow more accurate forecasting of AFC-30 funding needs for preventive maintenance.

i. <u>Replacement of Health Care Equipment</u>. Chapter 8 Section D of this Manual provides direction on how to obtain replacement of health care equipment. An effectively managed planned equipment replacement program minimizes repair costs and avoids loss of critical equipment at unscheduled times. Additionally, used but still serviceable equipment can be used by other facilities by "turn-in and reissue" through the Defense Reutilization Management Office (DRMO). At least annually, normally during the budgeting process, review the preventive maintenance costs for each piece of health care equipment. When repair and maintenance costs for the year exceed 50 percent of the current replacement cost of the equipment, then a U.S. Coast Guard Health Care Equipment Request, Form CG-5211, U. S. Coast Guard Health Care Equipment Request should be submitted to the HSWL SC, through the supporting clinic, requesting replacement.

j. <u>Disposal of Unserviceable or Outdated Medical Material</u>.

   (1) <u>Equipment and Supplies</u>. Property Management Manual, COMDTINST M4500.5 (series) provides guidance on when a formal survey is required. In general, a formal survey is not required except when equipment has been lost or stolen. If uncertain about whether or not a formal survey should be done, the unit's supply officer should be consulted.

   (2) <u>Pharmaceuticals and Medicinals</u>. Destruction of pharmaceuticals and medicinals will rarely be required. When disposal is necessary it must be done in accordance with federal, state, and local laws as well as applicable CG policy, if any (e.g. AVIP, SVP).

      (a) Prime Vendors provide a partial credit for some materials returned to them. IDHSs and supporting clinics will establish local policy for transfer of expired or short shelf-life pharmaceuticals. A transfer and replacement of pharmaceuticals within 6 months of expiration should be made with the supporting clinic to minimize waste.

      (b) If destruction is required, it will be accomplished in a well-ventilated area. Liquid substances present potential exposure through splash back. At a minimum, splash proof goggles and neoprene rubber gloves will be worn when working with liquid substances that may be absorbed through the skin. The wearing of protective equipment such as a splash apron is also encouraged. Thorough hand washing after the destruction process must be accomplished. Medical material must be disposed of in a manner so as to ensure that the material is rendered non-recoverable for use and harmless to the environment. Destruction must be complete, to preclude the use of any portion of a pharmaceutical. Chapter 8 Section C of this Manual provides detailed information about destruction and disposal of unsuitable medications.

k. Disposal of Medical Waste. Federal regulation defines how medical waste must be stored and disposed of, and the records that must be kept to document the storage and disposal. The information in the following paragraphs is provided as a general explanation of program requirements rather than an in-depth instruction on handling of medical waste. Medical waste must be classed in one of two categories: potentially infectious or non-infectious waste. In-depth guidance about storage, disposal and required record keeping for medical waste can be found in Chapter 13 of this Manual, in Quality Improvement Implementation Guide (QIIG) 16, and in Chapter 5 of the Safety and Environmental Health Manual, COMDTINST M5100.47 (series). An additional source of information is the unit's hazardous material control officer. In general, the disposal and record keeping requirements for the waste depend on the category of the waste:

(1) Potentially infectious waste is defined as an agent that may contain pathogens that may cause disease in a susceptible host. Used needles, scalpel blades, ("sharps"), syringes, soiled dressings, sponges, drapes and surgical gloves will generate the majority of potentially infectious waste. Potentially infectious waste (other than sharps) will be double bagged in biohazard bags, autoclaved if possible and stored in a secure area until disposed of.

(2) Used sharps will be collected in an autoclavable "sharps" container. "Sharps" will not be clipped. Needles will not be recapped.

(3) An adequate supply of storage and disposal material (containers, bags, etc.) must be maintained to ensure availability even on a long or unexpected deployment.

(4) A medical bio-hazardous waste log must be established and maintained, and must be kept on file for a period of 5 years. The medical bio-hazardous waste log must include the following information:

(a) Date of entry.

(b) Type of waste.

(c) Amount (in weight or volume).

(d) Storage location.

(e) Method of disposal.

(f) Identification number (if required by the state regulating authority). If such a number is required, the authority will provide it.

Chapter 9. B. Page 18

(5) Non-infectious waste includes disposable medical supplies that do not fall into hazardous waste. Non-infectious waste will be treated as general waste and does not require autoclaving or special handling. It should be placed into an appropriate receptacle and discarded with other general waste.

8. Health Services Department Administration.

a. Required Reports, Logs, and Records. Clear, accurate record keeping is of paramount importance for the IDHS. The quality of care provided to the unit's crew is reflected in the thoroughness of record and log entries completed by the IDHS. During compliance inspections and customer assistance visits, the IDHS and the unit will be evaluated at least in part on the accuracy and completeness of the reports and records created and maintained by the IDHS. The following records will be maintained in the Health Services Division. They will be in book/log form and in sufficient detail, to serve as a complete and permanent historical record for actions, incidents and data.

(1) Health Services Log. A Health Services Division log will be maintained by the IDHS. This log is a legal document. Entries will be clearly written in a concise, professional manner. The log may be either hand written or prepared using a typewriter or word processor but must be kept on file in "hard copy" form. It is used to document the daily operation of the Health Services Division. Chapter 1.Section B. of this Manual provides the requirement for this log. At a minimum, it will contain the names of all individuals reporting to sickcall for treatment, inspections, inventories conducted, and the results of potable water testing (if required). The log will be signed daily by the IDHS. It is worth noting that the Health Services Log will provide the information used in the Binnacle List (see required reports in this Chapter and Chapter 6 of this Manual), so a complete record containing information required in the binnacle list as well as other information of interest will streamline preparation of the report. All protected health information in the log must be kept private and secure in compliance with the Health Insurance Portability and Accountability Act of 1996 (HIPAA).

(a) Training Log. See "Training" in this Chapter.

(b) Biohazard waste log. This log will contain information as provided in Chapter 13 of this Manual.

(c) Health Records. Health records will be maintained and checked for accuracy and completeness as outlined in Chapter 4 of this Manual. The Health Record Receipt, Form NAVMED 6150-7 will be used whenever a Health Record leaves the custody of the IDHS. A quarterly check using the unit's alpha roster will ensure that any oversight is identified in a reasonably timely manner. All records checked out and not returned shall be reported to the command. No health record is to be taken to the field. If necessary for deployment, a battle record will be made up consisting of the following at a minimum:

[1] One Chronological Record of Care, Form SF-600.

[2] A copy of the Medical Readiness Reporting system printout of Immunization and Medical Readiness records

[3] A copy of the Adult Preventive and Chronic Care Flow Sheet, Form DD-2766.

(2) Required reports. Numerous reports are required at various intervals. A brief explanation along with a reference is provided for those not mentioned elsewhere in this chapter. Additionally, the information is provided in tabular format at the end of this section.

(a) Binnacle List. The binnacle list is normally a part of the Health Services Department Log. It is a listing of the names of the members provided treatment and the duty status determination resulting from the treatment. The list must be kept daily and submitted to the command for review as directed by the CO. It is normally reviewed each week by the XO and signed by the CO.

(b) Disease Alert Reports. See Chapter 7 of this Manual for requirements.

(c) Inpatient Hospitalization Report. See Chapter 2-A of this Manual.

(d) Food Service Sanitation Inspection Report. (Required for units with food service facilities) See the Food Service Sanitation Manual and A-10-a-(2) of this Chapter.

(e) Potable Water Quality Discrepancy Report (when not using a community based water source) required by Water Supply and Wastewater Disposal Manual, COMDTINST M6240.5 (series) Chapter 2.N.2 when potable water quality fails to meet requirements or is suspect.

(f) Readiness Report. The IDHS will assist the command in ensuring the medical and dental readiness for the personnel in their AOR by providing monthly Medical and Dental Readiness reports to the command.

Table 9-B-2

Reports Required Weekly

Report Name	Format or Form Required	Reference	Frequency or Date
Binnacle List	Locally designed form	COMDTINST M6000.1 (series) Chap 1. Section B.	Compiled daily, submitted weekly (or as directed by command).
Food Service Establishment Inspection Report	CG 5145	COMDTINST M6240.4 (series) Chap 11.	

Table 9-B-3

Reports Required Quarterly

Report Name	Format or Form Required	Reference	Frequency or Date
Controlled Substances Audit Board	Perpetual Inventory of Narcotics, Alcohol and Controlled Drugs, NAVMED 6710/5	Chapter 10.B. of this Manual	5th working day of the month

Table 9-B-4

Reports Required "As Needed"

Report Name	Format or Form Required	Reference	Frequency or Date
Readiness Report	locally designed form	See Paragraph 2-f of this section.	Monthly (or as directed by command).
Injury Report for Not Misconduct and In-Line-of-Duty Determination	CG-3822	See Paragraph 10-c of this section.	As needed. See paragraph 9.c of this chapter
Disease Alert Reports	RCN 6000-4	See Chapter 7-B of this Manual	As needed
Inpatient Hospitalization E-Mail	E-mail	See Chapter 2-A of this Manual	As needed
Potable Water Quality Discrepancy Report		COMDTINST M6240.5 (series)	when potable water quality fails to meet requirements or is suspect
Report of Potential Third Party Liability	CG-4899	COMDTINST 6010.16 (series) and chapter 6 of this Manual	As needed
Emergency Medical Treatment Report	CG-5214	COMDTINST M16135.4 (series)	As needed

1. Search and Rescue (SAR) Operations. In order for SAR units to provide the necessary level of medical support during SAR operations, COs must ensure personnel are trained to provide lifesaving measures in adverse and austere environments. The IDHS ashore may be called upon to play an integral role in the training and certification of unit personnel in first aid and cardiopulmonary-nary resuscitation (CPR). IDHSs who are certified as a First Aid and CPR Instructor by one of the following organizations: American Red Cross, National Safety Council, or American Safety and Health Institute have the ability to positively impact local units by providing the required medical training to boat crewmembers {Note: Personnel who serve as boat crewmembers aboard CG small boats are required to be certified in First Aid and CPR by one of the

aforementioned organizations in accordance w with the Boat Crew Seamanship Manual, COMDTINST M16114.5 (series) and the U.S. Coast Guard Boat Operations and Training (BOAT) Manual, Volume II, COMDTINST M16114.33 (series)}.

2. Environmental Health. Environmental health program related activities make up a large percentage of the daily responsibility of the IDHS. The link between environmental health and mission accomplishment cannot be over-emphasized. From a military perspective, environmental health and environmental health related problems accounted for almost eighty percent of personnel losses during past conflicts in which the United States was involved. For the purposes of this chapter, environmental health encompasses the disciplines of preventive medicine, sanitation and occupational health.

   a. Environmental Health Program Components. An effective environmental health program requires the IDHS to have a working knowledge of a large number of unit systems and work processes. An aggressive program of inspection and observation is required. These include:

      (1) Environmental Health Inspection.

      (2) Immunizations and Prophylaxis. The IDHS will ensure that all personnel receive required immunizations in accordance with Immunizations and Chemoprophylaxis, COMDTINST 6230.4 (series) and other relevant Commandant policy. Commandant (CG-1121), HSWL SC, and NEPMUs can provide up to date information on immunization requirements, disease intelligence, and preventive medicine precautions required for vessels deploying to OCONUS ports.

   b. Safety. The IDHS must become familiar with the work processes that are on-going at the unit and be able to recognize when they are not being performed in the proper manner or with the proper materials. The IDHS should report any safety related findings to the unit Safety Officer.

   c. Accident Reports. The Administrative Investigations Manual, COMDTINST M5830.1 (series) contains a requirement that a Injury Report for Not Misconduct and In-Line-of-Duty Determination, Form CG-3822 be completed whenever an injury results in temporary or permanent disability. This report is referred to in the Physical Disability Evaluation System, COMDTINST M1850.2 (series) as an "Line of Duty (LOD) Report" and a requirement is made that it be completed for all initial medical boards involving or resulting from trauma. Since it is difficult to determine the outcome of a serious injury in the early stages of treatment, a Injury Report for Not Misconduct and In-Line-of-Duty Determination, Form CG-3822 (also commonly known as an "Accident Report") is usually completed in such cases. It is not necessary to complete an "Accident Report" for any and all injuries unless command policy dictates otherwise.

d. Hazard Communication. The Hazard Communication Program is a unit wide program. Each unit will have appointed a Hazardous Materials Control Officer with overall responsibility for carrying out the program. Safety and Environmental Health Manual, COMDTINST M5100.47 (series) and Hazard Communication for Workplace Materials, COMDTINST 6260.21 (series) contain in-depth information about this program. The IDHS must be aware of the program requirements and its impact on the operation of the Health Services Division. Additionally, the IDHS must know the location of the unit's central MSDS file and have immediate access to product information which may be needed to render proper treatment to exposed crewmembers. Computerized databases available on CD-ROM are acceptable for this purpose if the Health Services Division contains appropriate access to the information

e. Eyewash Stations. Eyewash stations will be located in any space or work area with strong potential for splashes to, or foreign body injury of the eye. Eyewash stations will be maintained in accordance with the station's manufacturer requirements. Eyewash stations shall be flushed weekly for 15 seconds and flushed and drained according to the recommendations of the biostat ingredient manufacturer used in the station. This interval is usually every six months. Eyewash stations will be "tagged" with a maintenance record tag and inspection or maintenance activities will be recorded when performed. Inspections of eyewash stations will be recorded in the Health Services Log.

C. Independent Duty in Support of Deployable Specialized Forces.

1. Introduction. An independent duty health services technician (IDHS) is a Health Services Technician (HS) assigned to a unit that has no attached Medical Officer (MO). The identification or term Independent Duty Health Services Technician, used in any form, only identifies those Health Services Technicians that have successfully completed one of the three recognized Independent Duty Training courses, i.e. the USCG Independent Duty Health Services Technician, USN Independent Duty Corpsman, or USAF Independent Duty Medical Technician courses. Assignment to independent duty is challenging. The role is one of tremendous responsibility and at times can tax even the most experienced HS's skill, knowledge and ability. Along with the increased responsibility and sometimes arduous duty comes the potential for personal satisfaction unsurpassed by any other job assignment. The Deployable Specialized Forces (DSF) provides waterborne and, to a lesser extent, shoreside antiterrorism force protection for strategic shipping, high interest vessels, and critical infrastructure. DSFs are a response force capable of rapid, nationwide and international deployment via air, ground or sea transportation in response to changing threat conditions and evolving Maritime Homeland Security (MHLS) mission requirements. An assignment to one of these units requires additional knowledge, skills, and physical abilities beyond that of a general duty HS as the DSF may be deployed to areas that pose a great hazard from armed conflict and Weapons of Mass Destruction (WMD) agents (nuclear, chemical, and biological) as well as specific health care needs due to lack of local medical support. .

2. Mission, General Duties and Responsibilities.

   a. Mission. The IDHS serving with a DSF unit is charged with the responsibility for ensuring the personnel of the DSF are qualified for deployment. They will provide routine independent duty level medical care plus WMD knowledge and treatment of traumatic (e.g. gunshot) wounds if deployed with the team. It is recognized that HSs assigned to DSFs may participate in the same basic tactical training as non-HS DSF unit members, thus necessitating close coordination between the Executive Officer (XO) and Designated Medical Officer Advisor (DMOA) to ensure that both medical and tactical training needs are met

   b. General Duties. HSs on independent duty perform the administrative duties and, to the extent for which qualified, clinical duties (See United States Coast Guard Regulations 1992, COMDTINST M5000.3 (series) and Section 1-B of this Manual.). They shall not attempt, nor be required to provide, health care for which they are not professionally qualified. They shall provide care only for AD personnel; however they may provide care to non-active duty patients on an emergency basis. The filling of prescriptions for other than AD personnel shall be strictly limited to emergency situations and to authorized stock on hand under the allowance list for the unit. They may, under the guidance in Chapter 10 of this Manual, establish non-prescription medication programs for eligible beneficiaries.

c. <u>Responsibilities</u>. The Commanding Officer (CO) is responsible for the health and medical/dental readiness of the crew of his/her command. The health services department is charged with advising the CO of conditions existing that may be detrimental to the health of personnel and for making appropriate recommendations for correcting such conditions. Meticulous attention to all details and aspects of preventing disease must be a continuing program. It is imperative that sanitation and preventive health practices be reviewed constantly in order that any disease promoting situation may be discovered immediately and promptly eradicated. In the absence of a permanently assigned Medical Officer (MO), the DSF's CO will designate the Executive Officer (XO) to have direct responsibility for medical matters when no medical officer is assigned to the unit. The role of the Independent Health Services Technician (IDHS) is to assist the command in maintaining the good health and medical/dental readiness of the crew. To accomplish this responsibility, the IDHS must be informed of planned operations and anticipate any operational demands resulting from such operations. To this end, the IDHS will consult and advise the command in all matters with potential to effect crew readiness or the health of personnel. Some of the duties of the IDHS include but are not limited to:

(1) Assessment and treatment of illness and injury. Hold daily sick call. Diagnose and treat patients within capabilities. When indicated, refer cases to facilities where Medical or Dental Officers are available or, if this is not practical, obtain help and advice by radio or other expeditious means.

(2) Prevention of illness and injury through an aggressive environmental health program. Such a program includes inspection of living and working spaces as well as food service and storage areas; food storage and handling practices; integrated pest management practices; potable water quality surveillance; and recognition and management of communicable diseases.

(3) Train DSF personnel in the Coast Guard's Tactical Combat Casualty Care Self-Aid / Buddy-Aid and Combat Life Saver (CLS) programs (per Tactical Medicine Manual, COMDTINST M16601.16 (series)) or any other required medical training to meet the mission of the unit.

(4) Security and proper use of Health Services supplies, material and property.

(5) Supply and logistics to ensure supplies, materials and equipment necessary to carry out the mission of the Health Services Department are obtained and maintained in sufficient quantity and condition to support the unit mission and operation.

(6) Health Services Department administration, maintenance and security of health records. Maintain health records as required by Chapter 4 of this Manual. Ensure that all treatment records and/or consults from outside

referrals are obtained and placed in the health record. In addition, ensure that each patient is notified of all physical exams, consultations, and diagnostic tests (e.g., pap smears, mammograms, biopsies, x-rays, etc.) performed at any facility prior to filing in the health record. Maintain the security and confidentiality of all medical/dental records, databases and any other protected health information.

(7)   Maintenance and documentation of medical and dental readiness of unit personnel. The IDHS will assist the command in ensuring the medical and dental readiness for the personnel in their AOR by providing monthly Medical and Dental Readiness reports to the command, CGBI, scheduling the crew for required readiness exams and procedures as needed, and informing the command when a given crew member or department fails to cooperate with the IDHS's efforts to comply with readiness requirements. The IDHS shall also maintain a tickler system to include all return appointments requested by physicians or dentists from outside referrals requested by the command

(8)   Strict adherence to Chapters 1 and 2 of this Manual, which contain information about general and specific duties of the HS serving independently, including all required training on compliance with HIPAA privacy and security.

(9)   Other duties as assigned by the CO. In accordance with Paragraph 7-5-4, United States Coast Guard Regulations 1992, COMDTINST M5000.3 (series), HS may not be detailed to perform combatant duties in their own defense or protection of the wounded and sick in their charge, which are not prohibited by the Geneva Conventions. However, under routine situations; HSs who bear arms forfeit the special protections for medical personnel afforded by the Geneva Convention.

3.   Chain Of Command. The IDHS will normally be assigned to the Administrative Department and will report directly to the XO.

4.   Operation of the Health Services Department. The DSF Health Services Department is classified as a 1-D (ashore) sickbay. The unit may request a waiver from maintaining the full allowance list. This request will be routed through the assigned DMOA to the HSWL SC for approval. The IDHS is tasked with a wide variety and high volume of duties and responsibilities. This section sets forth policy and guidelines designed to assist the IDHS in carrying out assigned duties and responsibilities.

a.   Health Services Department Standard Operating Procedure. In order to successfully manage the Health Services Department, the IDHS must use time management and organizational skills and tools. One such tool is a written Standard Operating Procedure (SOP) for the Health Services Department. The SOP will govern the activity of the IDHS and has as its guiding precept the goals and missions of the unit. The SOP will be developed and submitted in written form to the CO for approval via the chain of command. In addition, the SOP will be reviewed at least annually by the IDHS, DMOA, XO and CO. The approved SOP will be kept in the Health Services Department for easy referral. Copies of pertinent sections will be posted as appropriate. The SOP will include:

(1) A copy of the IDHS's letter of assumption of duties as Health Services Department Representative.

(2) A copy of the HSs prescribing formulary approved by the DMOA.

(3) A written daily schedule of events for both on base and deployed periods.

(4) Copies of all letters of designation, assignment, and authority that directly impact upon the IDHS or Health Services Department. Examples include those granting "By direction" authority, designation as working Narcotics and Controlled Substances custodian, written certification to provide immunization (see Chapter 7 Section C) and assignment of a DMOA.

(5) A copy of the unit's organizational structure. This document will show graphically the IDHS's chain of command.

(6) A listing of duties and responsibilities assigned to the IDHS and the frequency that they are to be carried out. The listing will include both primary and collateral assigned duties.

(7) A listing of all required reports, the format required for submission, the frequency or date required, required routing and required "copy addressees". Incorporation of this information in tabular format provides a quick and easy guide for reference purposes.

(8) Guidance on how any change in a member's duty status is relayed from the member through the HS to the XO.

(9) A unit instruction or SOP for the management of rape or sexual assault cases. The document must provide policy for Health Services Department action in such cases, names of organizations, points of contact and telephone numbers for local resources as well as contact information for agencies and facilities which must be notified. CGIS must be notified on all **unrestricted reports** of alleged rape or sexual assault. It must contain a prearranged mechanism for timely completion of a physical examination by a **SAMFE or SANE** for the purpose of evidence gathering that meets requirements of all applicable law enforcement agencies. It must define limitations that will exist if the unit is deployed at the time the incident occurs. It must contain directions on how to complete a Victim Reporting Preference Statement, form CG-6095. **Additionally, it must define the unrestricted and restricted reporting procedures as outlined in the Sexual Assault Prevention and Response (SAPR) Program, COMDTINST M1754.10 (series).**

(10) A unit instruction or SOP for the management of suicide threat or

attempt. The document must provide policy for Health Services Department action in such cases, names of organizations, points of contact and telephone numbers for local resources, contact information for agencies and facilities which must be notified as well as a listing of required information, reports or actions.

(11) A unit instruction or SOP action required in the event of family violence. The document must provide policy for Health Services Department action in such cases, names of organizations, points of contact and telephone numbers for local resources, contact information for agencies and facilities which must be notified as well as a listing of required information, reports or actions.

b. Departure from the Daily Schedule of Events. The day-to-day operation of the Health Services Department is complex and impacted upon by the operational needs of the unit. It will of necessity change when events of higher priority or concern occur. If deviation from the daily schedule of events is required, notification to the chain of command will be made at the earliest opportunity. When deviation from daily schedule of events occurs frequently, the daily schedule of events will be reviewed and if necessary, changed. Any changes will be incorporated into the Health Services Department SOP and approved by the Commanding Officer.

c. Relief and Assumption of Duties as the IDHS. Proper documentation of the status of the Health Services Department and the condition of its equipment, stores, and records is required at the time of relief and assumption of the duties and responsibilities as the IDHS. This must be completed in order to adequately ascertain the state of operational medical readiness of the health services department and advise the local command. Operational readiness refers to the immediate ability to meet all health care demands within the unit's capabilities. The process is complex and requires both the incoming and outgoing IDHS to jointly perform the following:

(1) A complete inventory of all medical stores, spaces, and equipment, including durable medical equipment. Obtain the unit Health Services Allowance List and inspect the inventory of all health services department equipment, supplies, and publications. Initiate action for repair, survey, or replenishment of equipment, supplies, and publications. Verify inventory records and check all logs. Report any discrepancies to the local command without delay. Amplification of requirements and procedures is contained in Chapters 8 and 10 of this Manual

(a) A controlled substances inventory must be done. Use direction provided in Chapter 10 of this Manual.

(b) A complete inventory of all unit property in custody of the Health Services Department if the HS is the custodian of the property shall be conducted.

(2) A review of ongoing actions affecting the status of Health Services, e.g., outstanding requisitions, survey or repairs, and proper documentation of all such transactions.

(3) A review of the Health Services Department SOP.

(4) A review of the most recent HSWL SC Quality Improvement Assistance and Deployable Operations Group Ready for Operations Surveys for the unit. A copy of the surveys annotated with any finding of incomplete or uncorrected discrepancies will be included as an enclosure to the letter of relief.

(5) A review of all health records for completeness, accuracy, privacy and security. Check health records against the personnel roster. Any missing records should be accounted for or requested from previous duty stations. If records cannot be accounted for within one month's time, open a new health record. Check health records for completeness, and if not current, obtain and enter all missing information to the fullest extent possible. (See Chapter 4 of this Manual for further instructions pertaining to health records.)

d. <u>Letter of Relief and Assumption of Duties</u>. Upon completion of the Health Services Department review, a memorandum will be prepared and submitted by the oncoming IDHS via the chain of command and will advise the Commanding Officer of the status of the Health Services Department. A copy of the letter will be forwarded to the HSWL SC Senior IDHS Team Leader. The letter of Relief and Assumption of Duties will provide the following:

(1) Date of assumption of duties; a statement that the duties and responsibilities of the IDHS have been assumed; and that a thorough review of the Health Services Department has been conducted. Any discrepancies of material or record keeping will be annotated on a copy of the unit's most recent HSWL SC Quality Improvement site survey and submitted as an enclosure to the letter of Relief and Assumption of Duties as IDHS.

(2) Any discrepancies noted upon relief will be handled as a matter of individual command prerogative. Responsibility for correction, adjustment of account or inventory records, action required to replace missing items, as well as any necessary disciplinary action will be determined by the command.

(3) In cases in which no "on site" relief occurs, all of the preceding action will be completed. The supply officer of the unit will participate in the review process in place of the outgoing IDHS.

e. <u>Actions upon Proper Relief</u>. Upon assumption of duties as the unit's IDHS, one of the first tasks to complete is a thorough review of all SOPs and department instructions. Check the references; make contact with any listed points of contact. If possible, make visits and introductions in person. Find out how each system works and how it is accessed.

5. <u>Providing Health Care</u>. Delivery of health care is undoubtedly the most challenging and rewarding part of the job of any IDHS. The IDHS assigned to a DSF will have the challenges of having to deliver this care, at times, in remote locations during deployments as well as ensuring that any medical condition is evaluated to determine a member's status for deployment. This section is intended to provide a brief summary of the various facets of providing this medical care.

   a. <u>Designated Medical Officer Advisor (DMOA)</u>. Each DSF HS shall be assigned a DMOA. in accordance with Chapter 1 of this Manual. Good communication between the IDHS and the unit DMOA can prevent many problems affecting health care delivery to the crew. The IDHS will schedule a visit to the DMOA as soon as is practical after reporting aboard or upon completion of IDHS training. The purpose of the visit is to allow first-hand communication of expectations, support facility requirements, and any unique needs or concerns. This visit will normally be scheduled for a period of at least two weeks. This will allow the time required for the DMOA to evaluate the HS's performance factors and qualifications, and to develop a formulary for the HS. Open communication can be maintained through regular visits when practical, or at minimum, regular telephone calls. With regard to provision of direct care, the IDHS will seek DMOA or another MO's advice whenever there are questions about a patient's condition or when the following conditions exist:

      (1) Return to sick call before assigned follow-up because of failure to improve or condition has deteriorated.

      (2) Member cannot return to full duty status after 72 hours duration because of unresolved illness or injury.

      (3) The IDHS shall contact the Flight Surgeon on call through the closest Coast Guard Command Center when any of the following emergency conditions exist:

      (4) Undetermined fever of 102 degrees Fahrenheit or higher (when taken orally) persisting for 48 hours.

      (5) Fever of 103 degrees Fahrenheit or higher (when taken orally).

      (6) Unexplained pulse rate above 120 beats per minute.

      (7) Unexplained respiratory rate above 28 breaths per minute or less than 12 breaths per minute.

      (8) Depression with or without suicidal thoughts.

      (9) Change in mental status.

      (10) Chest pain or arrhythmia.

      (11) Unexplained shortness of breath.

      (12) Rape or sexual assault.

b. <u>Gender Considerations</u>. Chapter 1 Section B of this Manual provides specific direction for health services technicians about patient privacy, same gender attendant requirements, and examination restrictions.

c. <u>Avoiding Common Problems</u>. Scheduling and obtaining the routine medical care needed by crewmembers during non-deployed times can tax the organizational skills of even the most experienced IDHS. There are, however, actions that the IDHS can take which will enhance the chances of getting the routine appointments needed for all members. Some of these are:

(1) Identify the routine medical and dental needs of the crew. The DSF's supporting clinic has an established appointment scheduling procedure within which the IDHS must work whenever operational schedules allow. Follow the supporting clinics requirements for scheduling all appointments. When routine medical or dental care is to be made directly at a DoD MTF, the IDHS must determine the facility requirements for referral of patients and follow any local procedures.

(2) Communicate with the supporting clinic. Discuss the crew's medical and dental needs with the clinic supervisor and DMOA (if located at the facility).

(3) Perform all preliminary tests and complete all necessary paperwork before scheduling physicals at the supporting clinic.

(4) Post a listing of appointment dates and times as soon as it becomes available. Provide each Department/Division Chief a listing of the appointments applicable to the division or shop.

(5) Hold members accountable to be at their appointed place and time. Provide feedback to division officers and shop chiefs on any appointment failure. Notify XO of more than one failure.

d. <u>Consultations</u>. During the management of complex or protracted cases, consultations or specialty referral may be necessary. When such services are needed, the IDHS will normally make referral to a Coast Guard clinic, or in some cases, a Department of Defense medical treatment facility (DoD MTF). When referring a patient to see a Medical Officer at a CG health services clinic, the IDHS shall ensure that a Chronological Record of Care, Form SF-600 entry is completed using the SOAP format and that an appointment is scheduled. The clinic will normally provide treatment or arrange care if treatment is beyond its scope. When consultations or referral for specialty care are made directly to a DoD MTF, the IDHS must determine the facility requirements for referral of patients and follow any local procedures. Referrals to a DoD MTF will normally be documented using an Consultation Sheet, SF-513or a Referral for Civilian Medical Care, Form DD-2161. The consultation will provide a concise history of the condition to be evaluated as well as any pertinent findings. A provisional diagnosis is normally expected by the consultant. Chapter 4 Section B of this Manual provides direction on completion of a Consultation Sheet, Form SF-513. The patient and the patient's supervisor must be informed of all consultation or referral appointment dates and times. Courtesy is an important part of maintaining good working relationships with the facilities that the independent duty HS accesses for consultation and referral. Timely notification to the referral facility when appointment changes or cancellations occur (along with a brief explanation of why the change is required) helps maintain those relationships. Whenever possible, provide at least 24 hours notice for changes or cancellations.

e. Antibiotic Therapy. The IDHS may prescribe and administer antibiotics included on the Health Services Allowance List. The IDHS should consult with their DMOA or other Medical Officer for a recommendation or concurrence prior to administering antibiotic therapy. If consultation is not possible prior to administration, electronic notification, via email or message, must be sent to the DMOA providing case history, ICD9CM code and treatment provided.

f. Health Services Treatment Space. The Health Services treatment space will be manned at all times when patients are inside. All items are to be stowed in their proper place and secured. All medical records shall be locked in a cabinet. At no time should the Health Services space be left unlocked when the IDHS is not in the space.

g. Convalescent Leave/Sick Leave. Convalescent leave/Sick leave is a period of leave not charged against a member's leave account. It can be a recommendation to the command when a patient is Not Fit For Duty (usually for a duration expected to be greater than 72 hours) and whose recovery time can reasonably be expected to improve by freedom from the confines of quarters. It should be considered only when required as an adjunct to patient treatment. The command must evaluate each recommendation. Commands are authorized to grant convalescent leave as outlined in Military Assignments and Authorized Absences, COMDTINST M1000.8 (series).

h. Controlled Substances. Regulations for the handling, storage, and issue of narcotics and controlled substances are found in Chapter 10 of this Manual. The contents of this section are not intended to contradict the guidance provided there. This section serves to amplify policy provided with respect to medicinal narcotics and controlled substances as they pertain to the DSF. Narcotics and controlled substances require special handling. All controlled substances shall be obtained through the unit's collateral duty pharmacy officer.

(1) The CO will designate a commissioned officer as the controlled substances custodian (CSC). The CSC will follow the accounting procedure provided in Chapter 10 of this Manual. The IDHS will normally be assigned as custodian for narcotics and controlled substances working stock. Such assignment must be made in writing.

(2) All issues from working stock will be documented with a properly completed, written prescription. All non-emergent care requires contact with a Medical Officer before dispensing any controlled medication. The Medical Officer's orders will be documented on a prescription and in the patient's health record. The words "By verbal order of" will precede the ordering Medical Officer's initials, last name, time of order, and date of order both on the prescription and in the patient's health record. In the event of a true emergency, a Medical Officer's order is not needed to dispense a controlled substance. Once the emergency situation is over or alleviated, the IDHS will contact a Medical Officer, detail the circumstances and the controlled substances that were administered. Upon concurrence by the Medical Officer, the prescription prepared for the patient will be annotated with the words "By concurrence of" the ordering physician's initials, last name, time of concurrence and date of concurrence.

(3) The XO will countersign all prescriptions prepared by the IDHS prior to issue of any controlled substance or narcotic.

(4) Controlled substances shall be limited to amounts in the Health Services Allowance List for a 1-D unit. If the need exists for the unit to carry additional quantities of controlled substances based on use or potential for operational need, a written request signed by the Commanding Officer will be forwarded to the HSWL SC through the unit's DMOA. The request must include nomenclature, quantity, and brief justification.

i. Dental. It is the duty of the IDHS to arrange for the necessary dental examinations of the crew. All personnel should be Class I or Class II prior to deployment and all personnel must receive an annual dental exam and results must be documented in DENCAS.

j. Rape or Sexual Assault. **All victims of rape or sexual assault must be treated in a professional, compassionate, and non-judgmental manner. The unit shall have a SOP for cases of alleged rape and sexual assault. Refer to the Sexual Assault Prevention and Response (SAPR) Program, COMDTINST M1754.10 (series) for further guidance on reporting and responding.**

k. Suicide Prevention. An encounter with a suicidal person is always a deeply emotional event. It is important for the IDHS to act in a caring and professional manner. Early intervention and good communication skills are essential. If suicidal ideation is suspected it is important to remember:

(1) Take all threats and symptoms seriously. Immediately seek professional help from the nearest MTF for any member considering suicide. At no time should the person be left unattended. Once the patient is safe, contact the servicing Work-Life office for additional help or refer to Suicide Prevention, COMDTINST 1734.1 (series).

(2) Actively listen to the patient. Do not argue, judge, attempt to diagnose, or analyze the person's true intentions. It is important to provide a calm, caring, professional demeanor throughout the entire situation. Thoroughly document the patient encounter using the SOAP format.

(3) Arrange for an escort and a driver to transport the patient to the nearest Coast Guard clinic, DoD MTF or civilian emergency room with facilities appropriate to the situation. The unit's SOP for suicide threat or attempt should contain this information for ready use if needed.

l. Decedent Affairs. Chapter 5 of this Manual contains guidance about action that the Health Services Department must take when there is a death of a Coast Guard member. Military Casualties and Decedent Affairs, COMDTINST M1770.9 (series) contains further guidance concerning casualties and decedent affairs. It is unlikely that the IDHS will be assigned as the Casualty Assistance Calls Officer (CACO) for the command, but the IDHS will undoubtedly be heavily involved with the process of proper disposition of remains, so familiarity with the information required is helpful. The IDHS should also perform the following:

(1) An entry in the Health Services Log will be made detailing all available information concerning the death.

(2) The health record of the deceased member will be terminated in accordance with Chapter 4 of this Manual.

m. Disposition of Remains. As soon as possible, remains will be transferred to the nearest Military Treatment Facility (MTF) for further disposition. When transfer cannot be accomplished immediately, the remains will be placed into a body pouch and refrigerated at a temperature of 36 to 40 degrees Fahrenheit to prevent decomposition. The space must contain no other items and must be cleaned and disinfected before reuse. Remains will be identified with a waterproof tag, marked with waterproof ink, and affixed with wire ties to the right great toe of the decedent and also to each end of the body pouch. The minimum information needed on each tag includes the full name, SSN and rate or rank of the decedent. Whenever possible, do not remove items attached to the deceased at time of death. Such items may include (for example) IV lines, needles, AED pads, ET tubes, lengths of cord or line, etc. These may be important during an autopsy. Additionally, do not discard or launder clothing of the deceased. These items are sometimes important to surviving family members and in some cultures contribute to the mourning process of the deceased. This is a cultural consideration but should be a part of the decision process.

    n.   <u>Physical Disability Evaluation System</u>. The medical board process is detailed in Military Separations, COMDTINST M1000.4 (series) and the Physical Disability Evaluation System, COMDTINST M1850.2 (series).

6. <u>Training</u>. The purpose of training for both the assigned HS and that provided to the crew includes: assurance that the HS and crewmembers are able to provide aid for themselves and their shipmates in an emergency or a tactical/combat situation; and to promote the general health and well being of the crew.

    a.   <u>Training for the DSF HS</u>. In addition to the requirements of the rate, the HS will attend all general DSF training required of members of the DSF. In addition to this general DSF training the DSF HSs must successfully complete certain "C" schools is required. These are:

        (1) Coast Guard Independent Duty Health Services Technician School, Navy Surface Forces Independent Duty Technician School or the Air Force Medical Services Craftsman School.

        (2) Coast Guard Introduction to Environmental Health or Navy Basic Shipboard Series. (Note: This is not required for graduates of the CG IDHS School or Navy Surface Forces Independent Duty Technician).

        (3) Emergency Medical Technician - IDHSs assigned to deployable units are required to maintain currency with the National Registry of Emergency Medical Technicians (NREMT) at the EMT level. Short Term Training Requests are to be completed in accordance with the Training and Education Manual, COMDTINST M1500.10 (series) and forwarded to Commandant (CG-1121). Funding will be provided by Commandant (CG-11). See the Emergency Medical Services Manual, COMDTINST M16135.4 (series) for additional information. (This is part of the CG IDHS School).

        (4) Tactical Combat Casualty Care Live Tissue Training. The specific course and funding is to be determined by Commandant (CG-1121).

        (5) Instructor courses (must maintain current certification) in CPR, BLS, AED and First Responder

        (6) Field Management of Chemical and Biological Casualties course. HSs assigned in support of DSFs must complete this training. Funding will be provided by Commandant (CG-1121).

        (7) Recognition and Treatment of Dive Injuries. HSs assigned to DSFs that support dive operations must complete this training. Funding will be provided by Commandant (CG-11).

    b.   <u>IDHS Initial Certification</u>. All newly assigned IDHSs will participate in an orientation and certification program at their supporting clinic. Initial orientation must be completed within 60 days of reporting in to the new unit.

If due to operational commitments the orientation and certification cannot be completed within 60 days of reporting, a waiver request must be sent in memo format to the HSWLSC, SIDHS Team Leader. If the unit is unable to fund the TDY, the IDHS shall request funding from their HSWL SIDHS. Initial orientation and certification is estimated to take 2 weeks. During this time, the IDHS will:

(1) Work with his/her DMOA to complete the IDHS Operational Integration Form, CG Form 6000-4.

(2) See a minimum of 12 patients

(3) Perform a focused exam on each of the body's systems while using the DMOA as a guide and evaluator.

(4) Discuss with his/her DMOA notification procedures for the dispensing of scheduled drugs, administration of emergency medications and antibiotics.

(5) Solicit documented feedback from the DMOA and work to improve any areas where required.

(6) Perform a minimum of 4 clinical hours with a dental preceptor.

(7) Solicit documented feedback from the dental preceptor and work to improve any areas where required.

(8) Demonstrate a verbal understanding of management of acute dental problems to include dental abscess, periodontal disease, temporary fillings, fractured teeth, etc.

(9) Demonstrate documentation requirements for dental problems.

c. IDHS Annual Sustainment Training Requirements. Every 12 months, the IDHS must complete the following task:

(1) See a minimum of 48 patients/year. The IDHS shall solicit feedback from his/her DMOA on the patients treated over the last year.

(2) Work with his/her DMOA to complete the IDHS Operational Integration Form, CG Form 6000-4.

(3) Instruct at least one BLS certification class.

(4) Review all CEUs acquired over the last year in order to maintain EMT certification with his/her DMOA

d. Health Services Department Training Plan. A plan for training of the crew will be established in written form and kept on file. It will be based on a minimum 12 month cycle and be included in the unit training schedule. At a minimum, the following training will be given:

(1) Basic first aid.

(2) Shock, hemorrhage control, dressing.

(3) Airway management and assisted ventilation.

(4) Use of items in Individual First Aid Kits.

(5) Personal and dental hygiene.

(6) STI/HIV prevention.

(7) Heat and cold stress programs, including hypothermia.

(8) Respiratory protection program.

(9) Hearing conservation.

(10) Sight conservation.

(11) Blood borne pathogens.

(12) Additionally, at least one member of each boat crew will be trained as a Combat Lifesaver.

e. <u>Documentation of Training</u>. Documentation of the training is a requirement. An outline must be prepared and kept on file for all training topics presented and a training log maintained for all training provided. The training log will contain a record of all HS training given to the crew. It will contain the following information:

(1) Date.

(2) Topic.

(3) Duration.

(4) Instructor's name.

(5) Names (signatures of those present) of members trained.

f. <u>Training Format</u>. Training will normally be presented in either lecture format or demonstration and practical application. Lecture format presentations should be limited to 15 to 20 minutes and demonstrations and practical application should not exceed 1 hour. Practical application must be of high priority in training the crew in first aid, casualty evaluation, and treatment. There is no substitute for "hands on" practice in developing effective first aid skills.

7. <u>Supply and Logistics</u>.

a. <u>Custody of Health Services Equipment and Material</u>. As directed by the Commanding Officer, the IDHS is responsible and accountable for the health services material onboard the unit. As such, the IDHS is the custodian of all health service equipment and material. The custodian will not permit waste or abuse of supplies or equipment and will use techniques such as stock rotation, planned replacement and preventive maintenance to minimize waste of resources.

b. Inventory. An accurate record of medical stores and equipment must be maintained. The inventory of medical stores, spaces and equipment will be prepared using the NAVSUP-1114, Stock Record Card Afloat or in line item form (computerized database such as the IDHS inventory tool is an approved and preferred alternative if all necessary information is captured) and include:

(1) Quantity and shelf-life of each item currently on board.

(2) Balance on hand, high-level, low-level (reorder point for each item).

(3) Manufacturer, lot number and expiration date (pharmaceuticals).

(4) Quantity placed on order, date received.

c. Unit Property. Unit property in Health Services Department custody must also be safeguarded and accounted for. The unit property custodian should be contacted before transfer or destruction of such property.

d. Funding and Account Record Keeping. Funds used to purchase supplies and equipment, and to pay for the various expenses of operating the unit are broken down into Allotment Fund Control code (AFC) expenditure categories. This method allows for efficient budgeting and accounting. Fund categories generally used by IDHSs fall within the AFC subhead 30 or 57 expenditure categories.

(1) AFC-30 is a general unit fund used by the supply department to purchase generally needed operating supplies and services. Examples include pens, paper, books, training aids, etc. AFC-30 funding can be used to pay for Health Services Department supplies and equipment not obtainable through Defense Supply Center Philadelphia Prime Vendor Program (via the unit's supporting clinic) or the major medical equipment request process (see Chapters 6 and 8 of this Manual). Restrictions exist on what may be purchased with AFC-30 funds. Unit supply personnel can answer specific questions.

(2) AFC-57 is a funding category used to purchase health care related supplies and equipment, and to pay for health care. AFC-57 funds are distributed to the HSWL SC and further allocated by them to the units within their areas of responsibility with HS's assigned.

(3) With the full implementation of the Prime Vendor programs for Pharmaceuticals and for Medical and Surgical Supplies, AFC-57 fund allocations will be made to the Prime Vendor ordering point assigned for the unit.

e. Budgets and Budgeting. In general, IDHSs do not need to plan and submit an

AFC-57 budget request because medical supplies and equipment funding are controlled by the HSWL SC and Prime Vendor ordering points. If additional AFC-57 resource needs are anticipated, the IDHS's supporting clinic should be contacted for direction on how the resources are to be requested. The budget build process does have value for the IDHS however. AFC-30 funds will need to be planned for and requested and medical equipment in need of planned replacement must be identified and a Health Care Equipment Request, Form CG-5211 submitted. The budget build process is a good way to handle these needs. AFC-30 fund budget planning is relatively straight forward, although it can be time consuming. AFC-30 expenditures for Health Services should be broken into general use categories. Examples of categories are books and publications, non-consumable goods and services such as hydro testing and replacement of oxygen cylinders, and travel for continuing education. Budgeting categories can be as simple or complicated as the IDHS desires to make it. Once categories have been established, a ledger for the Health Services Department should be "opened" and the expenditure categories entered into it. The use of a "spreadsheet" program is an efficient way to keep an accounting record, but a ledger book works just as well. Attention to detail is the key. In general, a system using four to five categories works well.

(1) In preparing a budget for the upcoming year, it is important to look back over what was purchased in the previous year. To do this, collect all records of AFC-30 orders and expenditures. Review each line item and record the amount spent into the appropriate budget category. The steps for preparing a budget and carrying it out along with general timelines are contained in this paragraph. They are:

Table 9-C-1

March	Look back process. Review amount of funds spent over the first two quarters of the fiscal year as well as spending patterns for the previous fiscal year. Note general categories on which funds were spent and in which quarter items were ordered. This will allow projection of quarterly funding needs into the upcoming year.
April/May	Review status of the Health Services Department medical library and determine which texts and references must be updated. Review status of HS certifications and continuing medical education. Funding for training, conferences or seminars not normally funded by AFC-56 funds must be budgeted for as AFC-30 budget line items. Review preventive maintenance records and include cost projections in AFC 30 budget. Prepare and submit a Health Care Equipment Request, Form CG-5211 for medical equipment to be replaced. Seek guidance from XO on known or planned activities outside normal operations.
June	Submit finalized budget proposal through chain of command. AFC-30 budget information will be added to the unit budget. Be prepared to "defend" the budget request submitted. Documentation of the data gathering process and retrieval of the raw data used to justify the funding requested will likely be required. AFC-56 funds requests will be consolidated by the command and forwarded to the unit's district, HSWL SC or Area commander, as appropriate.

(2) Careful stewardship, good record keeping and accounting make existing funding and justification for increased funding levels easier.

f. Obtaining Pharmaceuticals, Medical and Surgical Supplies. Chapter 8 of this Manual provides policy applicable to the management of Health Services supplies. Prime Vendor programs for both Pharmaceuticals and Medical/Surgical Supplies have been established and it is through these programs that essentially all pharmaceuticals and supplies will be obtained. From an IDHS's perspective important aspects of the program include:

(1) Each unit has been assigned a Prime Vendor ordering point for Pharmaceuticals and for Medical/Surgical Supplies. The HSWL SC assigns the POCs and periodically updates the information. The Prime Vendor ordering point may be different for each of the programs.

(2) Funding for Prime Vendor for Pharmaceuticals and Prime Vendor for Medical/Surgical Supplies is provided to the assigned Prime Vendor ordering point by the HSWL SC. Internal accounting procedures vary among Prime Vendor ordering points. Some have established individual "accounts" for the units they are responsible for while others manage funds from a central account. Regardless of the accounting method used by the Prime Vendor ordering point, the IDHS must establish and maintain a system to track expenditures.

(3) Prime Vendor ordering points establish pharmaceutical and medical/surgical supply ordering procedures for their assigned units. Pharmaceutical and medical supply items ordered will be those required by the Health Services Allowance List (HSAL) in quantities required for the unit type. Deviation from the HSAL requirements will normally occur only after justification of the need is made by the IDHS to the DMOA for the unit. It will be made in writing and kept on file for review during HSWL SC site surveys.

g. Health Services Supporting Clinic. The supporting clinic for a DSF is the IDHS's partner in providing health care for the crew. Local agreements and resources may be available to allow the supporting clinic to provide a broader range of services to the IDHS and the crew but at a minimum, the following will be provided.

(1) All supplies and equipment (under $500.00) listed in the HSAL for the type of unit and on the HS Core Formulary. The unit no longer receives AFC-57 funding for the operation of the Health Services Department. These funds are provided instead to the supporting clinic with the intent that the supporting clinic will provide all required items for the IDHS to operate the Health Services Department.

(2) Assign the IDHS a DMOA in writing. The DMOA shall be available for questions about patient care, as well as completing record reviews quarterly.

(3) Perform medical boards for the IDHS unit as necessary.

(4) Provide a resource for advice and support in all administrative areas of health care delivery to include medical administration, physical examination review (within the approving authority of the Clinic Administrator), health benefits, medical billing and bill payment processing assistance, dental care, pharmacy administration, supply and logistics, bio-medical waste management, IDHS continuing education, and

quality assurance support. Any services provided at the clinic shall be extended to the IDHS to the maximum extent possible.

h. Preventive Maintenance of Health Services Equipment. Chapter 8 Section D of this Manual details the preventive maintenance program for Health Services equipment. An important part of medical equipment readiness is a program of preventive maintenance and planned equipment replacement. Repair and routine replacement part costs should be recorded on a locally generated form or side B of Medical/Dental Equipment Maintenance Record, CG Form NAVMED 6700. Capture of this data will allow more accurate forecasting of AFC-30 funding needs for preventive maintenance.

i. Replacement of Health Care Equipment. Chapter 8 Section D of this Manual provides direction on how to obtain replacement of health care equipment. An effectively managed planned equipment replacement program minimizes repair costs and avoids loss of critical equipment at unscheduled times. Additionally, used but still serviceable equipment can be used by other facilities by "turn-in and reissue" through the Defense Reutilization Management Office (DRMO). At least annually, normally during the budgeting process, review the preventive maintenance costs for each piece of health care equipment. When repair and maintenance costs for the year exceed 50 percent of the current replacement cost of the equipment, then a Coast Guard Health Care Equipment Request, Form CG-5211 should be submitted to the HSWL SC, through the supporting clinic, requesting replacement.

j. Disposal of Unserviceable or Outdated Medical Material.

(1) Equipment and Supplies. Property Management Manual, COMDTINST M4500.5 (series) provides guidance on when a formal survey is required. In general, a formal survey is not required except when equipment has been lost or stolen. If uncertain about whether or not a formal survey should be done, the unit's supply officer should be consulted.

(2) Pharmaceuticals and Medicinals. Destruction of pharmaceuticals and medicinals will rarely be required. When disposal is necessary it must be done in accordance with federal, state, and local laws as well as applicable CG policy, if any (e.g. AVIP, SVP).

(a) Prime Vendors provide a partial credit for some materials returned to them. IDHSs and supporting clinics will establish local policy for transfer of expired or short shelf-life pharmaceuticals. A transfer and replacement of pharmaceuticals within 6 months of expiration should be made with the supporting clinic to minimize waste.

(b) If destruction is required, it will be accomplished in a well-ventilated area. Liquid substances present potential exposure through splash back. At a minimum, splash proof goggles and neoprene rubber

Chapter 9. C. Page 19

gloves will be worn when working with liquid substances that may be absorbed through the skin. The wearing of protective equipment such as a splash apron is also encouraged. Thorough hand washing after the destruction process must be accomplished. Medical material must be disposed of in a manner so as to ensure that the material is rendered non-recoverable for use and harmless to the environment. Destruction must be complete, to preclude the use of any portion of a pharmaceutical. Chapter 8 Section C of this Manual provides detailed information about destruction and disposal of unsuitable medications.

k. Disposal of Medical Waste. Federal regulation defines how medical waste must be stored and disposed of, and the records that must be kept to document the storage and disposal. The information in the following paragraphs is provided as a general explanation of program requirements rather than an in-depth instruction on handling of medical waste. Medical waste must be classed in one of two categories: potentially infectious or non-infectious waste. In-depth guidance about storage, disposal and required record keeping for medical waste can be found in Chapter 13 of this Manual, in Quality Improvement Implementation Guide (QIIG) 16, and in Chapter 5 of the Safety and Environmental Health Manual, COMDTINST M5100.47 (series). An additional source of information is the unit's hazardous material control officer. In general, the disposal and record keeping requirements for the waste depend on the category of the waste:

(1) Potentially infectious waste is defined as an agent that may contain pathogens that may cause disease in a susceptible host. Used needles, scalpel blades, ("sharps"), syringes, soiled dressings, sponges, drapes and surgical gloves will generate the majority of potentially infectious waste. Potentially infectious waste (other than sharps) will be double bagged in biohazard bags, autoclaved if possible and stored in a secure area until disposed of:

(2) Used sharps will be collected in an autoclavable "sharps" container. "Sharps" will not be clipped. Needles will not be recapped.

(3) An adequate supply of storage and disposal material (containers, bags, etc.) must be maintained to ensure availability even on a long or unexpected deployment.

(4) A medical bio-hazardous waste log must be established and maintained, and must be kept on file for a period of 5 years. A medical bio-hazardous waste log must include the following information:

(a) Date of entry.

(b) Type of waste.

(c) Amount (in weight or volume).

(d) Storage location.

(e) Method of disposal.

(f) Identification number (if required by the state regulating authority). If such a number is required, the authority will provide it.

(5) Non-infectious waste includes disposable medical supplies that do not fall into hazardous waste. Non-infectious waste will be treated as general waste and does not require autoclaving or special handling. It should be placed into an appropriate receptacle and discarded with other general waste.

8. <u>Health Services Department Administration</u>.

    a. <u>Required Reports, Logs, and Records</u>. Clear, accurate record keeping is of paramount importance for the IDHS. The quality of care provided to the unit's crew is reflected in the thoroughness of record and log entries completed by the IDHS. During compliance inspections and customer assistance visits, the IDHS and the unit will be evaluated at least in part on the accuracy and completeness of the reports and records created and maintained by the IDHS. The following records will be maintained in the Health Services Department. They will be in book/log form and in sufficient detail, to serve as a complete and permanent historical record for actions, incidents and data.

        (1) <u>Health Services Log</u>. A Health Services Department log will be maintained by the IDHS. This log is a legal document. Entries will be clearly written in a concise, professional manner. The log may be either hand written or prepared using a typewriter or word processor but must be kept on file in "hard copy" form. It is used to document the daily operation of the Health Services Department. At a minimum, it will contain the names of all individuals reporting to sickcall for treatment, inspections, inventories conducted, and the results of potable water testing (if required). The log will be signed daily by the IDHS. It is worth noting that the Health Services Log will provide the information used in the Binnacle List (see required reports in this Chapter and Chapter 6 of this Manual), so a complete record containing information required in the binnacle list as well as other information of interest will streamline preparation of the report. All protected health information in the log must be kept private and secure in compliance with HIPAA.

        (2) <u>Training Log</u>. See "Training" in this Chapter.

        (3) <u>Biohazard Waste log</u>. This log will contain information as provided in Chapter 13 of this Manual.

        (4) <u>Health Records</u>. Health records will be maintained and checked for accuracy and completeness as outlined in Chapter 4 of this Manual. The Health Record Receipt, CG Form NAVMED 6150/7 will be used whenever a Health Record leaves the custody of the IDHS. A quarterly

check using the unit's alpha roster will ensure that any oversight is identified in a reasonably timely manner. All records checked out and not returned shall be reported to the command. No H/R is to be taken to the field. If necessary for deployment, a battle record will be made up consisting of the following at a minimum:

(a) One Chronological Record of Care, Form SF-600

(b) MRRS printout of Immunization and Medical Readiness records,

(c) Copy of completed Adult Preventative and Chronic Care Flowsheet, Form DD-2766.

b. <u>Required reports</u>. Numerous reports are required at various intervals. A brief explanation along with a reference is provided for those not mentioned elsewhere in this chapter. Additionally, the information is provided in tabular format at the end of this section.

(1) Binnacle List. The binnacle list is normally a part of the Health Services Department Log. It is a listing of the names of the members provided treatment and the duty status determination resulting from the treatment. The list must be kept daily and submitted to the command for review as directed by the CO. It is normally reviewed each week by the XO and signed by the CO.

(2) Disease Alert Reports. See Chapter 7 of this Manual for requirements.

(3) Inpatient Hospitalization Report. See Chapter 2-A. of this Manual.

(4) Food Service Sanitation Inspection Report. (Required for units with food service facilities) See the Food Service Sanitation Manual and Paragraph A-10-a-(2) of this Chapter.

(5) Potable Water Quality Discrepancy Report (when deployed and not using a community based water source) required by Water Supply and Wastewater Disposal Manual, COMDTINST M6240.5 (series) Chapter 2.N.2 when potable water quality fails to meet requirements or is suspect

(6) <u>Readiness Report</u>. The IDHS will assist the command in ensuring the medical and dental readiness for their personnel by providing monthly Medical and Dental Readiness reports to the command.

Table 9-C-2

Reports Required Weekly

Report Name	Format or Form Required	Reference	Frequency or Date
Binnacle List	locally designed form	COMDTINST M6000.1 (series) Chap 1. Section B.	Compiled daily, submitted weekly (or as directed by command).
Food Service Establishment Inspection Report	CG-5145	COMDTINST M6240.4 (series) Chap 11.	

Table 9-C-3

Reports Required Quarterly

Report Name	Format or Form Required	Reference	Frequency or Date
Controlled Substances Audit Board	Perpetual Inventory of Narcotics, Alcohol and Controlled Drugs, NAVMED 6710/5	Chapter 10.B. of this Manual	5th working day of the month

Table 9-C-4

Reports Required "As Needed"

Report Name	Format or Form Required	Reference	Frequency or Date
Readiness Report	locally designed form	See Paragraph 2-(g) of this section.	Monthly (or as directed by command).
Injury Report for Not Misconduct and In-Line-of-Duty Determination	CG-3822	See Paragraph 10-c of this section.	As needed. See Paragraph 9-c of this chapter
Disease Alert Reports	RCN 6000-4	See Chapter 7. Section B of this Manual	As needed
Inpatient Hospitalization Report	Message format	See Chapter 2. Section A of this Manual	As needed
Report of Potential Third Party Liability	CG-4899	COMDTINST 6010.16 (series) and Chapter 6 of this Manual	As needed
Potable Water Quality Discrepancy Report		COMDTINST M6240.5 (series)	When potable water quality fails to meet requirements or is suspect.
Emergency Medical Treatment Report	CG-5214	COMDTINST M16135.4 (series)	As needed

9. <u>Tactical Operations</u>. In order to provide the necessary level of medical support during tactical operations the IDHS and assigned DMOA will ensure that each team has personnel trained to provide lifesaving measures in adverse and austere environments. This can be accomplished by training one member of each operational team as a Combat Lifesaver. In addition the IDHS will train each member of the operational team in tactical Self-Aid/Buddy-Aid including the use of the hemostatic agent in the IFAK. The IDHS must also ensure the Combat Lifesavers maintain proficiency in their skills. The HS must also attend all aspects of operational training to ensure that they are prepared to respond with the team in

a high threat deployment where the CO feels the threat to the team requires a level of medical training above that of the regular team members.

10. <u>Environmental Health</u>. Environmental health program related activities make up a large percentage of the daily responsibility of the IDHS. The link between environmental health and mission accomplishment cannot be over-emphasized. From a military perspective, environmental health and environmental health related problems accounted for almost eighty percent of personnel losses during past conflicts in which the United States was involved. For the purposes of this chapter, environmental health encompasses the disciplines of preventive medicine, sanitation and occupational health.

   a. <u>Environmental Health Program Components</u>. An effective environmental health program requires the IDHS to have a working knowledge of a large number of unit systems and work processes. An aggressive program of inspection and observation is required. These include:

      (1) Environmental Health Inspection.

      (2) Immunizations and Prophylaxis. The IDHS will ensure that all personnel receive required immunizations in accordance with Immunizations and Chemoprophylaxis, COMDTINST 6230.4 (series) and other relevant Commandant policy. Commandant (CG-1121), HSWL SC and NEPMUs can provide up to date information on immunization requirements, disease intelligence and preventive medicine precautions required for vessels deploying to OCONUS ports.

   b. <u>Safety</u>. The IDHS must become familiar with the work processes that are on-going at the unit and be able to recognize when they are not being done in the proper manner or with the proper materials. The IDHS should report any safety related findings to the Safety Officer.

   c. <u>Accident Reports</u>. The Administrative Investigations Manual, COMDTINST M5830.1 (series) contains a requirement that a Injury Report for Not Misconduct and In-Line-of-Duty Determination, Form CG-3822 be completed whenever an injury results in temporary or permanent disability. This report is referred to in the Physical Disability Evaluation System, COMDTINST M1850.2 (series) as a "Line of Duty (LOD) Report" and requirement is made that it be completed for all initial medical boards involving or resulting from trauma. Since it is difficult to determine the outcome of a serious injury in the early stages of treatment, a Injury Report for Not Misconduct and In-Line-of-Duty Determination, Form CG-3822 (also commonly known as an "Accident Report") is usually completed in such cases. It is not necessary to complete an "Accident Report" for any and all injuries unless command policy dictates otherwise.

   d. <u>Hazard Communication</u>. The Hazard Communication Program is a unit wide program. Each unit will have appointed a Hazardous Materials Control Officer with overall responsibility for carrying out the program. The Safety and Environmental Health Manual, COMDTINST M5100.47 (series) and

Hazard Communication for Workplace Materials, COMDTINST 6260.21 (series) contain in-depth information about this program. The IDHS must be aware of the program requirements and its impact upon the operation of the Health Services Department. Additionally, the IDHS must know the location of the unit's central MSDS file and have immediate access to product information which may be needed to render proper treatment to exposed crewmembers. Computerized databases available on CD-ROM are acceptable for this purpose if the Health Services Department contains appropriate access to the information

e. Eyewash Stations. Eyewash stations will be located in any space or work area with strong potential for splashes to, or foreign body injury of the eye. Eyewash stations will be maintained in accordance with the station's manufacturer requirements. Eyewash stations shall be flushed weekly for 15 seconds and flushed and drained according to the recommendations of the biostat ingredient manufacturer used in the station. This interval is usually every six months. Eyewash stations will be "tagged" with a maintenance record tag and inspection or maintenance activities will be recorded when performed. Inspections of eyewash stations will be recorded in the Health Services Log.

D. <u>Quality Improvement Compliance Program</u> (QICP).

1. <u>Background</u>. The CG established an internal healthcare quality improvement (QI) program in the early 1990s to monitor the quality of healthcare delivered at its clinics and sickbays. The HSWL SC has historically administered the program by conducting QI surveys at each facility on a pre-determined schedule. However, in recent years the CG has moved to an external accreditation for its clinics, but sickbays are not subject to the accreditation program. The need for a QI program that ensures sickbay compliance with CG specific healthcare issues and health readiness still exists. CG specific QI and operational health readiness issues are monitored by the HSWL SC under the Quality Improvement Compliance Program (QICP).

2. <u>Purpose</u>. The intent of the QICP is to assist with and ensure all Independent Duty Health Services Technicians (IDHS) comply with and maintain CG specific healthcare-related requirements and unit operational health readiness.

3. <u>Overview</u>.

   a. <u>Definitions</u>.

      (1) Operational Readiness. Standards established by the CG that determine whether individual members and units are prepared to meet their assigned missions.

      (2) Quality Improvement. See Chapter 13 of this Manual.

4. <u>Program Elements</u>. The QICP is designed to monitor healthcare-related QI requirements for sickbays and to ensure units within their area-of-responsibility (AOR) are operationally ready in accordance with CG standards. Elements that are applicable in the QICP for sickbays are:

   a. Unit Demographics

   b. Administration

   c. Record Maintenance

   d. Fiscal and Supply Management

   e. Preventive Maintenance

   f. Health Care Delivery

   g. TRICARE

   h. Professional Education

   i. Pharmacy Services

   j. Environmental Health and Safety

   k. Operational Readiness

5. <u>Collaborative Program</u>. The primary mission of CG sickbays is to maintain the operational health readiness of active duty and reserve personnel by assuring their availability to physically and mentally meet worldwide deployment standards in accordance with the Medical Manual COMDTINST M6000.1 (series). Maintaining a high level of health readiness involves collaboration between providers, commands, clinics, sickbays and the HSWL SC.

6. <u>Monitoring the QICP</u>. It is the responsibility of the unit Independent Duty Health Services Technician to develop and maintain a plan that ensures optimal health readiness for all active duty/reserve members within the designated AOR in accordance with guidance provided in this instruction. The HSWL SC will review CG-specific QI and operational health readiness issues on a continual basis and provide needed assistance to sickbays to ensure a high level of health readiness. QI compliance will be accomplished through HSWL SC assist visits. A post-visit evaluation report will be provided to the unit CO through the Designated Medical Advisor Officer and supporting Clinic Administrator.

7. <u>Assistance Program</u>. The QICP is designed to provide an environment in which QI and operational health readiness of sickbays are monitored on a continuous, versus retroactive, basis. The QICP is an assistance program designed to ensure a high level of care is provided at CG sickbays and that a high level of operational health readiness is maintained. The program assists sickbays in meeting both CG readiness and QI standards.

8. <u>Responsibility</u>.

   a. HSWL SC.

      (1) Ensure the Commandant's Health Care QI Program is executed at the field level.

      (2) Ensure that Independent Duty Health Services Technicians (IDHSs) are performing their duties in strict adherence to this manual.

      (3) Conduct site visits on a two-year cycle (more often as defined by current certifications) to verify standards compliance and to provide assistance in meeting the expectations of the QICP.

      (4) Develop and maintain health services support program guides necessary to provide operational guidance for IDHS activities.

      (5) Develop and maintain Quality Improvement Self Assessment Checklists for assist visits.

      (6) Provide technical and professional advice regarding health services to units, as required.

      (7) Ensure the IDHSs Operational Integration Form has been filled out and signed by the IDHS and DMOA.

b. Units.

   (1) Ensure the unit actively pursues health services standards for independent duty as set forth in this manual and the HSWL SC Quality Improvement Compliance Program.

   (2) Develop and maintain a plan that ensures optimal health readiness for all active duty/reserve members within the designated unit AOR in accordance with guidelines provided in this instruction.

   (3) Continually monitor all sickbay QA activities by reviewing the HSWL SC QI Checklist.

9. QI Compliance Checklist. The compliance checklist shows QI and/or operational readiness tasks that sickbays must address on a regular basis. The checklist is used to assess compliance with Quality Improvement standards. There are *Basic Elements* and *Key Elements* that hold pre-determined weighted values and will allow the HSWL SC surveyor to assign the appropriate certification based on the compliance level. To view the most current QI Compliance Checklist, go to the following web site in CG Central: IDHS QI Checklist

10. Compliance Certification Standards. Because sickbays are not subject to an external accreditation, continued oversight by the HSWL SC is critical to ensure that IDHS's are performing all duties required of them. This oversight is achieved through site visits every 2 years. HSWL SC will designate the Regional Practice SIDHS to use the Compliance Checklist and evaluate the performance level of each IDHS site. A detailed report will be provided with a summary of any discrepancies or recommendations for improvement. Based on the result, the HSWL SC surveyor will determine the appropriate re-visit rotation as follows:

a. Full Certification: Full certification is obtained by achieving at least ninety percent (90%) for compliance. Sickbays in compliance with at least ninety percent (90%) of the key elements and at least ninety percent (90%) of the basic elements will be fully certified. Full Certification requires no re-visit and the certification is good for 2 years.

b. Provisional Certification: Provisional certification is given when a sickbay's compliance falls below 90%. Sickbays in compliance with at least eight (80%) of the key elements and at least eighty percent (80%) of the basic elements will be provisionally certified. A Provisional Certification requires a re-visit in 6 months or 1 year as determined by the surveyor.

c. Non-Certification: A Non-Certified status is given when a sickbay's compliance falls below 75%. Sickbays falling below 75% compliance will not be certified and require a 3-month follow-up assessment.

11. Post Survey. At the conclusion of a QI visit a Command out brief shall be conducted between the Regional Practice SIDHS & XO/CO to discuss the outcome of the visit. A detailed report describing all discrepancies and an Executive Summary outlining the findings and recommendations will be provided to the command no

later than 30 days following the date of survey. A written plan of corrective action shall be sent to HSWL SC within 30 days of receipt of the survey results. The plan shall be vetted through the assigned DMOA and address all items listed under the Summary of Pertinent Findings.

E. <u>Independent Duty Management of TRICARE.</u>

1. <u>Introduction.</u> The role of the Military Health System (MHS) is to enhance DoD and our Nation's security by providing health support for the full range of military operations and sustaining the health of all those entrusted to its care, which includes all active duty service members (ADSM). The MHS supports the military mission by fostering, protecting, sustaining and restoring health.

2. <u>Discussion.</u> The IDHS must be aware of the policies and concepts that surround the MHS. The MHS includes all Department of Defense Military Treatment Facilities (MTF), USCG Clinics, and the civilian network providers contracted by the Managed Care Support Contractors known as TRICARE providers. Depending on the location of your command, you may work with all of these entities in the coordination of primary and specialty health care for your crew.

3. <u>Access to Care.</u> There are four basic steps that will ensure almost seamless access to health care:

   a. The first step is a check-in process for new arrivals to your unit. Every member should be required to visit sick bay upon arrival.

   b. Second, each member must be properly enrolled to a PCM, either military or civilian, depending on your local policy. It is required by law (32CFR) and DOD/CG policy that all active duty personnel with a permanent duty assignment of 180 days or more enroll in a TRICARE Prime Program. The enrollment process requires the member to fill out a form and choose a Primary Care Manager (PCM). Enrollment forms can be obtained from the local TRICARE Service Center which typically are co-located with the MTF or can be found online at www.tricare.mil

   c. ADSMs are required to get all non-emergent health care from their PCM

   d. ADSMs are required to get pre-authorization for specialty care from their PCM.

4. <u>Access to Care Standards.</u> The MHS has specific access standards to care that are important for the IDHS to understand to ensure the crew is getting the appropriate care in a timely manner. It is important to note that the access standards for family members and retirees are slightly different. They are as follows:

   a. Urgent care appointment—24 hours or less

   b. Routine appointment—7 days or less

   c. Specialty appointment or wellness visits— Within four weeks or 28 days

   d. Travel time may not exceed 60 minutes from work to the PCM office.

e. Travel from ADSM's home for referred specialty care should not exceed 1 hour.

f. If the service is not available at the MTF within the appropriate access standards, beneficiaries should be referred to a TRICARE network provider if available.

5. <u>Enrollment</u>. Managing the crew's enrollment outside the catchment of a CG or DoD MTF. In this situation your crew will be enrolled into what is known as TRICARE Prime Remote (TPR).

6. <u>Resources</u>. It is important for the IDHS to understand that there are CG, DOD and TRICARE resources available to assist with challenges and issues both for the individual as well as systemic concerns regarding health care.

a. Beneficiary Counseling and Assistance Coordinator (BCAC). Located at all MTF locations as well at the HSWL SC. For the CG BCAC call 1-800-9-HBAHBA (1-800-942-2422). BCACs improve customer service and satisfaction, enhance beneficiary education troubleshoot complicated, delayed, and mishandled issues, and respond to phone, e-mail, and written correspondence

b. Debt Collection Assistance Officer (DCAO). Located at all MTF locations as well at the HSWL SC. For DCAO assistance call 1-800-9-HBAHBA (1-800-942-2422). The DCAO will assist with TRICARE-related collection (debt) problems, assist with negotiations with collection agencies, credit bureaus, and agencies, research the problem, and recommend appropriate actions to resolve the problem. Contact DCAO when a collection notice is received.

c. The Military Medical Support Office (MMSO). MMSO serves as the centralized Service point of contact (SPOC) for customer service and medical case management for all eligible Active Duty military and Reserve component service members within the 50 United States and District of Columbia. MMSO also coordinates all civilian health care services outside of the cognizance of a Military Treatment Facility for TRICARE Prime Remote (TPR). HSWL SC has a detached billet at the CG SPOC and can be reached at 1-888-647-6676, option 7 ext. 6716.

CHAPTER 10

PHARMACY OPERATIONS AND DRUG CONTROL

Section A. Pharmacy Administration.

Section B. Controlled Substances.

Section C. Forms and Records.

Section D. Drug Dispensing Without a Medical Officer.

CHAPTER TEN – PHARMACY OPERATIONS AND DRUG CONTROL

A. Pharmacy Administration.

1. Responsibilities.

a. Duties of designated person. The person designated in writing as responsible for the pharmacy is accountable to the Senior Health Services Office (SHSO), or the Executive Officer, for properly storing and dispensing drugs, record keeping, and maintaining a pharmacy policy and procedures manual, including HIPAA complaint privacy and security provisions, and ensuring limited access into the pharmacy during and after hours.

b. Responsibility. The person in charge of the pharmacy shall acquire, store, compound, and dispense medications according to applicable Federal laws (principally Title 42, United States Code and Title 21, Code of Federal Regulations and observe the highest standards of professional practice and established pharmaceutical procedures to ensure the best possible in patient safety and/or patient medication safety practices. This responsibility includes maintaining appropriate inventory and monitoring of expiration dates of all pharmaceuticals. Specific units have been/will be tasked by Commandant (CG-11) to maintain special stocks of pharmaceuticals. Quarterly, all units maintaining pharmaceuticals used for the purpose of anthrax prophylaxis or pandemic influenza prophylaxis are to provide summary data to the HSWL SC Pharmacy Officer to include name(s) of pharmaceutical agent, amount on hand, lot number, and expiration date. The HSWL SC Pharmacy Officer shall maintain this information and provide to Commandant (CG-11) when directed.

c. Pharmacy references. The person in charge of the pharmacy shall ensure adequate and appropriate current pharmacy references, hardbound and/or online access (e.g., Drug Facts and Comparison, a drug information handbook, a drug interaction reference, a drug identification reference, Sanford Guide to Antimicrobial Therapy, Mosby's Nursing Drug Reference, a pediatric dosage handbook, a drugs during pregnancy and lactation reference, etc.).

d. Request funding. Through medical administration, persons responsible for daily pharmacy operations shall request adequate funding to provide the level of pharmaceutical care required in Section 10.A.2.

e. Regional Pharmacy Executive Oversight. Regional Pharmacy Executive (RPE) collateral duty oversight shall be provided for all regional practice site locations and sickbays that do not have Pharmacy Officers assigned. The details of the Pharmacy Officer Collateral Duty Program are delineated in QIIG 45, which shall be administered by the HSWL SC, who shall:

(1) Determine cost requirements for the Pharmacy Officer collateral duty program and submit funding requests to Commandant (CG-112) in the annual operating summary of budget estimates process.

(2) Provide direction and funding to Pharmacy Officers for matters relating to assignments in pharmacy officer collateral duty program.

(3) Develop work plans specifying units for which the Pharmacy Officer is responsible.

(4) Ensure visit schedule will be:

    (a) The most cost effective.

    (b) Feasible to maintain responsibilities at the unit where the pharmacy billet is assigned.

    (c) Coordinated with the unit CO possessing the billet.

(5) Supervisors and those regional practice site commands desiring input into the Regional Pharmacy Executive's USPHS Commissioned Officers' Effectiveness Report (COER) are referred to the HSWL Supervisor's Guide for guidance and forms.

(6) Oversees the following responsibilities of collateral duty Pharmacy Officers who:

    (a) Report to the SHSO of the unit to which they are assigned.

    (b) Follow the established chain of command.

    (c) Serve as the secretary of the Pharmacy and Therapeutics Committee (PTC) for the regional practice.

    (d) Be responsible for all aspects of the Prime Vendor (PV) Pharmaceutical Program.

    (e) Assist each unit in eliminating or minimizing the purchase of medication through nonfederal sources by using formulary process and redistributing medication as needed.

    (f) Provide oversight to the Health Services Technician(s) who normally operate the regional practice site pharmacy and assist in dispensing operation as required.

    (g) Provide and document in-service training to the regional practice site staff. Provide and document all training provided to Health Service corpsmen (other than "C" school pharmacy trained technicians working with the pharmacist in the pharmacy), including those IDHS corpsmen at regional practice site locations.

    (h) Review all pharmacy operations and policies including controlled substance activities.

    (i) Assist the regional practice site in preparation of the pharmacy, and other areas of the practice site under the responsibility of the pharmacy, for AAAHC and HSWL SC Quality Improvement Surveys.

(j) Update quarterly information on the DoD Shelf Life Extension Program (SLEP), making it available to the CG SLEP Coordinator for submission to the HSWL SC Pharmacy Officer (op-m). For access to the SLEP website, information can be obtained at: https://slep.dmsbfda.army.mil/portal/page/portal/SLEP_PAGE_GRP/S LEP_HOME. Provide current information as provided in the Medical Material Quality Control (MMQC) messages. Pharmacies will document review of MMQC messages that contain information on medication recall or warnings and the appropriate actions taken as described in the message. Documents shall be retained for period of three years after which they be destroyed. Ensure messages include reviewer's initial, date of review and the action taken.

(k) Reference QIIG 45, Regional Pharmacy Executive (RPE) Area of Responsibility (AOR) Program, for additional guidance.

2. Prescribers.

   a. Authorized prescribers include:

   (1) Medical Officers and Dental Officers as defined in Sections 1.B.1. and 1.B.4. of this Manual.

   (2) Civilian medical and dental providers employed by the CG.

   (3) While performing isolated duty or underway, HSs may prescribe additional drugs listed in Health Services Allowance List Afloat, COMDTINST 6700.6 (series). HSs in these situations shall seek medical direction and advice from their assigned Designated Medical Officer Advisor (DMOA).

   (4) Civilian physicians, dentists, and allied health care providers (nurse practitioners, physician assistants, optometrists, etc.) as authorized by state law in their licensing jurisdiction to write prescriptions within the scope of their professional practice.

   (5) Uniformed service medical and dental officers/providers, other than CG, authorized by their service to write prescriptions within the scope of their professional practice.

   b. Non-clinic issued prescriptions. Prescriptions written by other uniformed services or civilian medical or dental officers/providers for formulary medications shall be honored at CG pharmacy locations where a registered pharmacist is physically present on site. If a registered pharmacist is not available, presented prescriptions will not be filled or dispensed. DoD prescription policies (i.e. TRICARE) shall be observed to the fullest extent possible within the scope of the primary care nature of CG Health Care facilities and based upon the DoD Basic Core Formulary (BCF). Prescriptions that are auto-opened, computer generated or electronically signed will NOT be accepted in CG pharmacy practice site locations. Prescriptions written for medications that are not included on the practice site formulary will be returned to the patient and the patient will be referred to a nearly Military Treatment Facility (MTF) or to the TRICARE prescription network.

c. Formulary medications. Prescriptions for eligible beneficiaries from licensed uniformed, civilian or outside physicians, dentists, or podiatrists shall be honored for products on the clinic's formulary provided a registered pharmacist is available on site. Regional practice site formularies are to be based on DoD BCF guidelines and the CG regional practice.

(1) For those CG clinics with a Pharmacy Officer permanently assigned, the BCF contains the minimum drugs that each pharmacy must have on its formulary and provide to all eligible beneficiaries.

(2) For those CG clinics without a Pharmacy Officer permanently assigned, there are no requirements to stock the entire contents of the BCF. Military practitioners or contract providers shall not countersign civilian/outside prescriptions nor shall civilian/outside prescriptions be rewritten during cursory outpatient visits with the intent of authorizing the prescription for dispensing at the facility.

(3) In the case of multiple strength BCF drugs, all strengths need not be stocked but all prescriptions for that agent will be filled, regardless of strength. Pharmacists shall use discretion to determine if the prescribed dose can be filled using the available strengths the pharmacy carries (e.g. hydrochlorothiazide 25 mg can be filled with 50 mg strength with pharmacy instruction on the label to read "take ½ tablet").

(4) If additional funding is required for specific, high cost drugs, it shall be requested via the AFC-57 budget process via the HSWL SC.

(5) For CG patients referred out of the practice site for specialty care: Patients shall be advised by their referring CG provider that prescriptions written by the consulting provider may be filled at the CG practice site pharmacy location where the consultation was generated IF the medication prescribed is included on the practice site's formulary. Prescription written may, also, be filled at a DoD MTF pharmacy, or through the TRICARE prescription network (retail or mail order). After completion of the patient's consultant appointment, patients shall return to the referring CG provider with the consultation brief, maintaining the continuity of care and assessment of the treatment plan.

d. Self Prescribing. Authorized prescribers shall not prescribe controlled medications for themselves and/or their family members. If such medication is required and no other authorized prescriber is assigned to the regional practice site or sickbay, the CO, or XO, shall review, approve, and countersign each controlled prescription before it is filled by pharmacy personnel.

3. Prescriptions.

   a. Prescriptions written by CG providers. Prescriptions written by CG providers shall be filled at the facility where written. In cases of emergencies where it is advisable for a patient to start a prescription immediately and it is not available at the pharmacy, prescriptions may be written on a Prescription Form, DD-1289 or other approved prescription blank (s) so that the patient may have the prescription filled through the TRICARE prescription network (retail or mail order). Prescriptions written by Health Services Technicians shall be filled only at the practice site facility where written. CG practice sites may agree amongst themselves to honor another CG regional practice site's provider prescriptions if stock shortages so necessitate. Other CG facilities may honor CG physician assistants' and nurse practitioners' refills (for other than controlled substances) if the patient presents his or her health care record containing the original entry.

   b. Telephoned and verbal prescriptions. At the Pharmacy Officer's discretion, telephoned and verbal prescriptions may be accepted only in emergencies. CG clinics without a Pharmacy Officer shall not accept telephone prescriptions.

   c. Facsimile prescriptions. At the Pharmacy Officer's discretion, faxed prescriptions may be accepted. Faxed prescriptions for controlled/narcotics will NOT be accepted. CG regional practice sites without a registered pharmacy officer will not accept faxed prescriptions under any circumstances.

   d. Transferring prescriptions. Prescriptions may be transferred at the discretion of the Pharmacist. The transferring of prescriptions shall only be conducted between licensed Pharmacists. If a licensed Pharmacist is not available, patients shall be requested to obtain a new prescription. ONLY a one time transfer of the same prescription number is authorized. Multiple transfers of the same prescription number are not authorized.

   e. Contacting providers. Health Services Technicians shall not contact civilian/outside prescribers to resolve prescription problems but shall return the problem prescription back to the patient and explain the reason the prescription cannot be dispensed. The HS may provide a copy of the regional practice's formulary for reference if the reason for the unacceptable prescription is that the medication is not included on the practice site's formulary.

   f. Prescriptions shall be personalized. If more than one member of a family is prescribed the same drug, a separate prescription shall be generated for each member.

   g. Scope of practice. Items prescribed must treat conditions within the normal scope of prescriber's professional practice and the ethics of the prescriber.

   h. Cosmetic conditions. Prescriptions for medications to treat cosmetic conditions (baldness, wrinkles, etc.) or for weight loss will not be honored nor shall these medications be stocked at CG practice site facilities.

i. <u>Prescriptions for animals</u>. Prescriptions for animals other than Government owned shall not be filled.

j. <u>CG Provider</u>. If a CG provider has clinical privileges at a local DoD facility, he or she may use its prescription form to write prescriptions to be filled at that facility, provided the form contains the statement "To be filled only at [insert designated DoD facility]."

k. <u>Special order medications</u>. Special order medications will not be ordered at CG regional practice sites for dispensing. Medications dispensed at regional practice sites will be those medications that are included in the CG regional practice site formulary. Patients receiving a prescription for a medication that is not on the practice site formulary will be referred to the TRICARE prescription network.

4. <u>Prescribing in the Medical Record</u>.

a. <u>Process</u>. The CG method of prescribing for Medical Providers is the Provider Graphic User Interface (PGUI) and Point of Entry (POE) as per Chapter 14 of this Manual. At all regional practice sites and sickbays, patient medications will be ordered by utilizing the Chronological Record of Care, Form SF-600 or when appropriate an Emergency Care and Treatment, Form SF-558. The medical record thus becomes a more comprehensive repository for all patient health information and ensures the pharmacy staff has access to the necessary clinical information (age, weight, allergies, laboratory values, vital signs, etc.). In the case of dental care, Dental Providers shall write prescriptions in the dental record on Dental Record Continuation, Form SF-603A. For controlled prescriptions written by Dental Providers, a single hard copy of the prescription (e.g., Prescription Form, DD-1289) is required as well. For medical providers utilizing PGUI or POE or controlled substances an additional Prescription Form, DD-1289 is not required. However for proper documentation and accountability of the controlled substance, the Pharmacy Staff will generate a duplicate pharmacy label of the ordered controlled substance medication, placing it on a prescription blank. The patient shall sign the back of this "generated prescription" with the appropriate documentation as designated in the Coast Guard Medical Manual, COMDTINST M6000.1 (series), Chapter 10-B.6.b.4.

b. <u>Procedures</u>.

(1) Documentation shall be subjective, objective, assessment and plan (SOAP) format, notating the patient visit on a Chronological Record of Care, Form SF-600 or Emergency Care and Treatment, Form SF-558 in the chart. Under the "Plan" section, the drug name, strength, directions, quantity, and refills will be listed. Prescriptions shall be legibly written. Abbreviated names of medications and unapproved acronyms shall be avoided to prevent medication errors and enhance patient safety.

(2) In the "Plan" section, state a disposition to assist pharmacy staff in coordinating quantities of all chronic medications until the next

appointment. Complete the entry with the authorized prescriber's signature.

(3) The terms chronic and maintenance medications are synonymous. A maintenance medication is defined as any medication used to treat a chronic condition. The term "maintenance" implies that a prescriber and patient have gone through a dosage titration process and have determined that the patient should be "maintained" on an effective dose of a medication that is well tolerated. Ultimately, the individuals in a position to make such a determination are the patient and the prescriber. The standard quantity issued for chronic conditions is a 90-day supply. If it is necessary to deviate from this amount, prescribe quantities in 30-day increments (30, 60, 90, etc.) if possible. If pharmacy personnel in consultation with the prescriber, deems it advantageous to the patient due to travel, deployment, operational commitments, packaging, etc., they may dispense larger quantities (up to 180 days). Active Duty members deploying outside the continental United States (OCONUS) for greater than 180 days will be instructed to use the TRICARE Mail Order Program (TMOP).

(4) For in-house prescriptions and prior to dispensing, in the event of a medication error, incomplete entry, or question/concern regarding a medication, pharmacy staff shall contact/notify the prescriber for further guidance. Upon confirmation/clarification from the prescriber, completely draw a single horizontal line through errors or changes and conspicuously write "Error" next to the item. The person changing the entry shall initial the change or error. If the provider requires further review before making a change, return incorrect or incomplete entries to the prescriber for revision/review. The medication error shall be documented in a Medication Error Report.

(5) Pharmacy personnel will adhere one-part of the multi-part strip of the prescription label that designates the patient name, drug, and quantity on the PGUI or POE generated Chronological Record of Care, Form SF-600 and all members will initial in ink to signify who prepared the prescription (i.e., the member filling the prescription and the member checking the prescription). For refills, a prescription log or book shall be established and utilized. The pharmacy staff will adhere one-part of the multi-part strip of the prescription label that states the patient name, drug, and quantity in the log or book and all members will initial the label in ink to signify who prepared the prescription (i.e., the member filling the prescription and the member checking the prescription).

(6) Pharmacy staff shall write the manufacturer's name, lot number, and expiration date to the right of the drug prescription (not required with CHCS). Sickbays not utilizing CHCS shall maintain a drug dispensing log, containing prescription number, patient's name, patient's SSN, drug name, drug manufacturer, lot number and the medication's expiration date. This log shall be retained for 3 years.

(7) In addition to the Chronological Record of Care, Form SF-600, or Emergency Care and Treatment, Form SF-558, entry, written prescriptions are required for all prescriptions (including controlled substances) in the event a prescription must be taken to another MTF pharmacy facility or through the TRICARE prescription network for dispensing. When controlled substance prescriptions are processed in-house, documentation shall be separated, maintained and filed appropriately (i.e., CII file and CIII-V file) by pharmacy staff and retained in the pharmacy.

(8) All prescriptions generated from sources other than the regional practice site shall be filled or re-filled using the CHCS system and maintained on file in the pharmacy. For patients utilizing the regional practice site pharmacy services only and not maintaining a health care record at the facility will be offered the HIPAA MHS Notice of Privacy Practices. Pharmacy personnel shall ensure DEERS eligibility with every prescription visit.

(9) At regional practice sites where a Pharmacy Officer/Pharmacist is available, the Pharmacy Officer/Pharmacist shall make a significant effort to ensure all prescriptions are double-checked by a pharmacist, prior to dispensing to the patient. At regional practice sites where the Pharmacy Officer/Pharmacist is unavailable, the RPE may allow a "C" school trained pharmacy technician to prepare and dispense prescriptions. Recommendation is made for the "C school trained pharmacy HS technician to be double checked by another "C" school pharmacy trained HS technician, ensuring an extra level of patient safety. At practice sites where neither a pharmacist nor a "C" school pharmacy trained technician is available, corpsmen that have completed the Watchstander qualification (QIIG 41.1) may on a TEMPORARY BASIS, but not more than 6 months, prepare and dispense prescriptions that have been double checked (with appropriate MO document) by the medical provider at the local regional practice site.

5. Signatures. No prescription order shall be filled unless it bears the signature of an individual authorized to write prescriptions. All prescriptions shall include the printed or stamped name, rank, and professional discipline (MD, DDS, HS2, etc.) of the prescriber. Prescriptions for controlled substances shall also provide the NPI or DEA number of the prescriber. Pharmacy personnel shall maintain signature examples for in-house and contract prescribers. Professional judgment shall be used to verify authenticity of prescriptions that are generated from a source other than an in-house CG provider.

6. Dispensing.

a. The pharmacy shall serve as the source of supply from which regional practice sites or satellite activities normally obtain required pharmaceuticals and related supplies. In addition, the pharmacy dispenses medications and preparations as authorized directly to patients.

b. Prescription verification. Except for approved non-prescription program items, the pharmacy/sickbay will dispense all stocked items only on receiving a properly written, verified prescription or an in-house computer generated prescription. If the pharmacy staff receives an illegible prescription or questions its authenticity, dosage, compatibility or directions to the patient, clarification from the prescriber will be obtained prior to the dispensing the medication(s).

c. Medication recall. Regional practice sites and sickbays shall have a system (computerized, written, etc.) in place to ensure that prescriptions can be retrieved in the event of a product recall and be able to segregate the recalled product until additional guidance is provided.

d. Adverse medication reaction reporting. Regional practice sites shall submit patient adverse reactions or product quality problems via the FDA MEDWATCH system on FDA Form 3500, which can be obtained from the FDA at 1-800-FDA-1088 or at the FDA website: www.fda.gov. Vaccine Adverse Event Reporting System (VAERS) forms can also be obtained at the same website.

e. Patient identification. When dispensing medication(s) to patient(s), the dispenser shall identify the patient through a military identification card and ensure DEERS eligibility.

f. Medication information. Pharmacy personnel shall ensure patients receive a printed copy of the medication's patient education monograph with all new prescriptions that accompanies the CHCS generated prescription label. Additionally, FDA required Medication Guides that are currently not included in the patient education monograph shall be made available to the patient. These can be obtained from the FDA website at http://www.fda.gov/Drugs/DrugSafety/ucm085729.htm.

g. Medication Error. In the event of a medication error (i.e. an error discovered after a prescription has been dispensed to the patient), a Pharmacy Error Report including pertinent information relevant to the error (name of discoverer, date of discovery, a brief statement describing error, and steps taken to prevent recurrence) shall be completed. A copy of the report shall be submitted for review during the next convening Regional Practice Pharmacy and Therapeutics Committee (PTC) meeting and a copy of the completed PTC meeting minutes will be forwarded for review and inclusion in the minutes of the next convening Regional Practice Quality Improvement Focus Group meeting.

h. Medication containers. Child-resistant containers shall be used to dispense all prescription legend medications except sublingual nitroglycerin tablets, which are to be dispensed in the original packaging. The prescribing provider or the patient may specifically request a conventional (non-child resistant) closure. When the request is generated by the provider, the prescription order will be indicated accordingly. If the patient requests such a closure, a statement on the backside of the prescription will be notated and the patient will sign and date the annotation. In the case where a patient is requesting ALL of his/her prescription to be dispensed with a conventional closure, the pharmacy personnel will ensure that a signature card is generated, containing the statement: "I request non-childproof closures for all medications prescribed for me", is completed, signed and dated by the patient. Signature cards shall include the date, printed name of the patient, initials of the pharmacy staff assisting the patient and shall be maintained at the pharmacy location until the patient permanently leaves the area or has not used the facility within one year of the original date of the signature card. The patient's CHCS profile shall be annotated in the Pharmacy Patient Comment (PPC) to reflect the patient's request.

i. Refills. Prescriptions (except for controlled substances, see Chapter 10-B-4.c.) may be refilled when authorized by the prescriber. The maximum quantity of medication authorized for refills shall be for up to a one (1) year supply of medication. No prescriptions shall be refilled after more than one (1) year from the date it was written. PRESCRIPTIONS SHALL NOT BE REFILLED FROM THE CONTAINER LABEL. Verification of an ongoing prescription order shall be verified in the CHCS system before a refill is dispensed to the patient.

j. Non-prescription Medication Program. CG regional practice sites are encouraged to establish non-prescription medication programs under the following guidelines:

(1) CG regional practice sites/sickbays with assigned health care personnel may elect to operate a nonprescription drug program. Units not staffed with an HS may operate a nonprescription medication program with oversight provided by a CG RPE or supporting IDHS. Units electing to offer the CG non-prescription drug will obtain authorization through the HSWL SC Pharmacy Officer and will verify that they will operate within the established CG non-prescription program guidelines.

(2) All CG regional practice sites/sickbays shall make condoms available to beneficiaries even if the location does not elect to offer the CG non-prescription medication program. Condoms shall be made available to beneficiaries under the age of 18 years unless specifically forbidden by law.

(3) Items available shall be limited to those medications specifically identified (authorized) in the CG non-prescription medication program (Figure 10-A-1). Practice sites may elect to offer a limited selection of authorized products to their patients, but shall NOT add unauthorized products (even if the product is classified as over-the-counter in the retail sector). All products must be dispensed in the manufacturer's FDA approved packaging with the mandated instructions and warnings. Locally packaged items are not authorized.

(4) A beneficiary family shall be limited to a maximum of two (2) items per week from the CG non-prescription medication program.

(5) Items shall be available ONLY during normal operating hours of the pharmacy or the sickbay.

(6) Pharmacy or sickbay personnel shall monitor the non-prescription medication program for perceived overuse/abuse. Individuals suspected of this misuse shall be referred to a medical provider for assessment and may have access to this privilege terminated.

(7) The CG non-prescription medication program items shall not be dispensed to pregnant patients or non-active duty beneficiaries under 18 years of age. Local flight surgeons shall determine which of the program's products may be acquired by aviation personnel.

(8) Regional practice sites offering the CG non-prescription medication program will maintain monthly statistics for the quantity of items provided to beneficiaries. This figure shall be separated from regular pharmacy workload statistics and will not be tallied as a part of the practice site's number of prescriptions. The quantity of items provided on the non-prescription medication program will be an additional statistic provided to the health service administrator (HSA). Only those prescription medications that have been dispensed by written prescription orders shall be counted in the practice site's total number of prescriptions. Once non-prescription medications forms have been collected and tallied, the request forms may be shredded, except for those requests for products containing pseudoephedrine, which will be retained for three (3) years.

(9) To receive an item from the CG non-prescription medication program, patients must sign a log or complete a request form which certifies the following:

(a) I do not wish to see a physician or other health care provider for advice before receiving these medications. I understand that the medication is for minor illness or conditions and that if symptoms worsen or persist longer than 48 hours, the person for whom this medication is intended should be seen by a health care provider.

(b) I am not pregnant or under 18 years of age (unless active duty). If on flight status, I understand that I am only authorized to receive over-the-counter items approved by the Flight Surgeon.

(c) The person for whom this medication is intended does not have high blood pressure/cardiac problems, diabetes, thyroid problems, and is not taking blood thinners.

(10) Individuals suspected of returning for medication for a non-resolving problem shall be referred to a medical provider for evaluation. In addition, beneficiaries requesting medical advice that in the opinion of the pharmacy or sickbay personnel is beyond their expertise shall be referred to the medical provider.

(11) The log sheet or request form shall contain the current date, patient's name and quantity of the item(s) received. For medication containing

pseudoephedrine, in addition to the above required items, the patient address shall be included on the designated log sheet or request form.

(12) Pharmacy personnel shall ensure positive control and a tracking mechanism for any items on the CG non-prescription medication program list, containing pseudoephedrine. Pharmacy personnel shall ensure that all beneficiaries, requesting any items on the non-prescription medication program, containing pseudoephedrine have signed the request form prior to dispensing. These request forms shall be segregated from the other non-prescription medication program request forms and maintained in the pharmacy for a period of three (3) years.

(13) Funding for independent duty HS (IDHS) assigned units that will offer the CG non-prescription medication program shall acquire funding of the products from their district regional practice's AFC-57 account.

(14) Figure 10-A-1 provides a sample form for the non-prescription medication program with a current list of authorized items.

k. At larger regional practice sites where a night locker/locked cabinet is utilized and, in such situations when the pharmacy is closed, a medical or dental officer, or other authorized person, shall dispense medication(s) only from the locked vehicle, which contains pre-packaged medications in limited supply for "after-hours" dispensing. The locked cabinet shall contain a small supply of medications that are typically required to treat acute medical conditions. Prescriptions generated from sources outside of the CG practice site shall not be filled after regular pharmacy operating hours. In these situations, patients will be advised of alternative resource availability.

l. A sign shall be posted outside of the pharmacy practice site in a highly visible location stating "Please inform our pharmacy staff if you are breast feeding or may be pregnant."

m. Pharmacies shall adhere to the TRICARE guidance of the mandated dispensing of generic medications.

n. Drug samples are not authorized at CG regional practice sites/sickbays.

o. For guidance on pharmaceutical gifts, the CG Ethics Program can be found in Standards of Ethical Conduct, COMDTINST M5370.8 (series), specifically Chapter 2-C.

7. Labeling.

a. Requirements. A label will be prepared for each prescription dispensed to individuals and will be securely affixed to the container prior to dispensing. The label or appropriate auxiliary labeling will show as a minimum:

(1) Facility identity, including the pharmacy address and telephone number.

(2) Consecutive identifying number.

(3) Prescribers name.

(4) Definitive, concise directions to the patient.

(5) Drug name and strength.

(6) Quantity dispensed.

(7) Patient's first and last name.

(8) Inked initials of person preparing the prescription label and the person double checking the prepared prescription.

(9) The legend "KEEP OUT OF THE REACH OF CHILDREN" on all prescription labels.

(10) Date prescription filled.

(11) Refill status.

(12) Expiration date for prepared and compounded prescriptions (e.g. liquid antibiotics, dermatologic products, etc.).

(13) The legend "CAUTION: FEDERAL LAW PROHIBITS THE TRANSFER OF THIS DRUG TO ANY PERSON OTHER THAN THE PATIENT FOR WHOM IT WAS PRESCRIBED" (for controlled substances only).

(14) Necessary supplemental or auxiliary labels.

b. Directions on labels. If prescription contents are for external use only or require further preparation(s) for use (shaking, dilution, temperature adjustment, or other manipulation or process) include the appropriate directions on the label or affix an additional label to the container. If liquid preparations for external use are poisonous, affix a "poison" label to the container. If medicines prescribed for internal use are poisonous, use sound judgment whether to label them "poison" based on the finished preparation's potency in each case.

c. Generic names. Medicinal preparations compounded or packaged in the pharmacy for subsequent issue will be identified and labeled with the full generic name. The manufacturer's name, lot number, and expiration date, if any, will be shown on the label.

d. Multiple Dose Injectables. All multiple dose injectable vials shall be dated upon opening. The expiration date will be reflected as twenty-eight (28) days from the opening of the product, except in situations where the manufacturer's product information indicates a shorter expiration date.

8. Drug Stock.

a. Source of medications. The Defense Logistics Agency (DLA) is the primary source of medications for either the "Depot" system or prime vendor contracts. Other Federal sources (Perry Point IHS Depot, Federal Supply Schedules, HSWL SC negotiated purchase agreements, etc.) may be used when medication is unavailable or the price/service advantages are determined to be the most cost effective procurement method for the regional practice site.

b. Nutritional/Herbal/Dietary Supplements/Medications and Performance Enhancing Substances. Scientific information (quality and production control, adverse effects, drug interaction, side effects) regarding these products are often times scanty or nonexistent. Many of these products have interactions with other medications in unpredictable ways, The possible/potential side effects from these agents are difficult to predict, occur with irregularity, interact differently in any body system and may affect the central nervous system, cardiovascular system, vision, balance, mood, behavior, learning and cognitive ability. Active duty personnel are required to be operationally ready, stand watch/post, and/or perform special duties. Due to the active duty personnel requirement to remain alert with full senses and reasoning capabilities, active duty members may neither possess, use, nor purchase (via any venue) herbal supplements, dietary products, or alternative health care substances banned or not approved by the FDA for sale or use in the United States. Only those items that have been licensed and approved by the Food and Drug Administration (with the exception of vitamins with an established RDA) are authorized for use. CG regional practice health care sites shall not purchase or dispense "herbal supplements" or "dietary supplements". Patients should inform their healthcare providers if they are taking any type of "supplement" to avoid potential drug interactions. Aviators and flight crew members shall follow guidance provided in the Coast Guard Aviation Manual, COMDTINST M6410.3 (series), Chapter 7. Commands can contact the RPE or the HSWL SC Pharmacy Officer for additional guidance.

c. Separation of dosage forms. For the storage of any medications stocked in the regional practice site pharmacy/sickbay, external use medications shall be separated from internal use medication and ophthalmic medications shall be separated from otic medications. Caustic acids such as glacial acetic, sulfuric, nitric, concentrated hydrochloric, or oxalic acid shall not be issued or stored in regional practice pharmacy/sickbays, but shall be stored in separate lockers, clearly marked as to contents. Methyl alcohol shall not be stored, used, or dispensed by the pharmacy.

d. Refrigerated items. Pharmaceuticals requiring refrigeration shall be stored within proper refrigeration equipment which meets the USP criteria for pharmaceutical storage. Refrigerators shall be installed with alarms and constant temperature monitoring and recording devices and shall be connected to an emergency power supply to protect refrigerated medications in the event of an electrical malfunction or power surge. Temperature readings will be checked and recorded twice daily. Temperatures which register outside the acceptable storage range will be immediately reported to the RPE, the HSA (if ashore) or the Executive Officer (if afloat). Refrigerated medications will be stored and maintained at a temperature between 36-46 degrees F. The HSWL SC Pharmacy Officer can be contacted for further guidance on resources for obtaining refrigerators and temperature monitoring devices. Vaccines shall not be stored in the same refrigerator used to store food as the potential increased access to the (food) refrigerator compromises the stable temperature environment for the vaccines. Additionally, the potential hazard of vaccines contaminated by food spill or spoilage could compromise the vaccine. Additional guidance can be found at: http://www.cdc.gov/vaccines/pubs/pinkbook/vac-storage.html#temperatures

e. Room Temperature items. Medications that are identified as requiring storage at room temperature will be maintained within a temperature range of 59-77 degrees F.

f. Hazardous substances. Store flammable drugs according to accepted fire safety regulations. Additional information regarding hazardous materials can be found at: http://www.uscg.mil/directives/ci/6000-6999/CI_6260_31B.pdf.

g. Doors. Solid core doors with one-inch (minimum), throw key-operated, dead-bolt locks shall be used for all pharmacy and medical supply areas and shall be secured at the end of the day. On Dutch doors, both sections shall have this type lock. Pharmacy doors shall have a second key lock or cipher lock to remain secured at all times.

h. Shelf Life Extension program. When eligible drugs are listed on the DoD FDA Shelf Life Extension Program (SLEP), the regional practice site's identified drug "to be tested" shall be removed from stock and labeled with project number until the results are received. Upon result notification, items shall be marked with FDA approval labels, which will contain the new expiration date and the medication shall be returned to stock. In the event that the medication expiration date is not extended, the drug shall be forwarded to the reverse distribution company for credit or disposal. The SLEP program determines the eligible medications that will be tested and are based upon the enrolled medications submitted by the SLEP participants.

i. Poison antidotes. The regional practice site pharmacy shall maintain, in the prominent practice site areas, an adequate supply of emergency medications and poison antidotes (the National Poison Control Center telephone number is 1-800-222-1222). Containers for these items shall be closed with break-away seals to prevent the unreported removal of items. The outside of the container shall display an inventory product list, including expiration dates.

9. Credit return program (Reverse Distribution Program). Regional practice site pharmacies/sickbays shall establish a credit return program through an approved pharmaceutical returns vendor that accepts expired pharmaceuticals and disposes of them in accordance with federal law. The company shall coordinate and issue refunds from the respective manufacturers of the returned products directly to the practice site's prime vendor account and the prime vendor will issue it as available credit for the specific practice site location. Expired medications not accepted by the returned goods vendor shall be disposed of as biohazard waste. DLA currently has an established contract with several reverse distribution or returned goods vendors. Participating facilities shall select from one of the contracted vendors, following guidance as provided by DLA. Prior to transfer of

medications to the returns vendor, pharmacy personnel shall ensure that a printed inventory of <u>all</u> returned pharmaceuticals will be prepared and retained at the pharmacy location BEFORE the pharmaceuticals are removed from the practice site location. Quarterly at the next scheduled PTC meeting, the RPE shall review returned pharmaceuticals data for trends that may indicate a need to modify inventory levels or ordering practices and make recommendations to the committee. If controlled substances are included in the pharmaceutical returns, pharmacy personnel shall ensure appropriate documentation has been completed, signed and retained (e.g., Requisition And Invoice/Shipping Document, Form DD-1149 and Perpetual Inventory, Form NAVMED 6710).

10. <u>Pharmacy and Therapeutics Committee (PTC)</u>.

    a. This is a mandatory advisory committee in all CG regional practice site health care facilities and will include all practice sites within the respective district, which have assigned medical officer and shall meet quarterly in a face-to-face, video or teleconference. The PTC will be conducted centrally as a function of the Regional Practice for that district and each clinic in the district will participate in the meeting. The committee is composed of, but not limited to, the following members and will constitute a quorum: the Senior Medical Executive (SME) or representative, the Senior Dental Executive (SDE) or representative, the Regional Pharmacy Executive (RPE), the Regional Practice Manager (RPM) or representative, and one representative from each clinic within the district. HSAs are strongly encouraged to attend. The chairman will be the SME and the RPE will be the secretary.

    b. The committee is an advisory group on all matters relating to the acquisition and use of medications. Recommendations made are subject to the approval of the SHSO. The basic responsibilities of this committee are to:

        (1) Use of the Department of Defense (DoD) Basic Core Formulary (BCF) will be the basis for the regional practice site formulary.

        (2) The regional practice site pharmacy's formulary will include medications and protocols as designed in the CG Standardized Health Services Allowance List (HSAL) formulary.

        (3) The regional practice site pharmacy formulary shall not include items based primarily on civilian prescriber demand.

        (4) Prevent unnecessary therapeutic duplications of formulary products.

        (5) A review of all non-formulary items the pharmacy procures and dispenses will be conducted. To meet this requirement, the regional practice PTC will review:

        (a) A list of all regional practice site pharmacy formulary items not currently in the DoD BCF.

        (b) A list of all special order items (Special Order Medication Request forms) and the patients for whom procured.

(6) Conduct an ongoing drug usage evaluation (DUE) program for selected medications.

(7) Monitor the regional practice site's controlled drug prescribing and usage.

(8) Review pharmacy policies and procedures, as necessary.

(9) Monitor the quality and accuracy of prescriptions and patient information the pharmacy provides and enacts any quality assurance measures deemed necessary.

(10) Reviews any adverse reaction or product quality reports (VAERS or MEDWATCH).

(11) Monitors compliance with HIPAA privacy and security mandates.

c. Documentation for upcoming PTC meetings will be forwarded to the RPE in the first month of each quarter for inclusion to the PTC agenda, which will be prepared and forwarded to the SHSO for approval prior to the meeting. The PTC meeting will be conducted in the second month of each quarter. Minutes of the meeting will be prepared and forwarded to the SHSO for approval by the end of the third month of the quarter and then returned to the RPE for retention and uploaded to the CG's online CG Portal Microsite. A copy of the minutes will be forwarded to the regional practice manager.

d. Quality Improvement Implementation Guide (QIIG) #5, Pharmacy and Therapeutics Committee provides additional guidelines.

Figure 10-A-1

CG REGIONAL PRACTICE SITE NON-PRESCRIPTION MEDICATION PROGRAM
USCG (may insert name of practice site or location here)
Limited to TWO (2) Items Per Family Per Week

This program is for military beneficiaries only. MILITARY ID CARD IS REQUIRED.
Please read and sign the following statement:

_____ I do not wish to see a physician or other health care provider for advice before receiving these medications. I understand that these medications are for minor illnesses or conditions and that if symptoms worsen or persist longer than 48 hours, the person for whom this medication is intended should be seen by a health care provider.

_____ I am not pregnant or under 18 years of age (unless active duty). If on flight status, I understand that I am only authorized to receive over-the-counter items approved by the Flight Surgeon.

_____ I will inform the pharmacy staff if the person for whom this medication is intended has high blood pressure, cardiac problems, diabetes, thyroid problems, is taking blood thinners.

Signature: _____

Printed name: _____Date: _____

Address:(Required only for products containing Pseudoephedrine)

_____

_____

NOTE: Items listed may be available.

__ Acetaminophen 325mg tabs, #50	___ Cetylpyridinium Anesthetic Loz, 30gm
__ Acetaminophen 80 mg chewable tabs, #30	___ Guaifenesin 100mg/5ml syp., 120ml
__ Acetaminophen 160mg/5ml liq., 120ml	___ Guaifenesin 100mg/DM 5mg/5ml syp., 120ml
__ Antichap, Lipstick	___ Diphenhydramine 25mg caps #24
__ Liquid Antacid, 150ml	___ Diphenhydramine 12.5mg/5ml liq., 120ml
__ Ibuprofen 200mg tabs, #24	___ Bacitracin oint., 15gm
__ Ibuprofen 100mg/5ml soln., 120ml	___ Analgesic Balm, 30gm
__ Pseudoephedrine 30mg tabs, #24	___ Clotrimazole Topical crm 15 gm
__ Saline Nasal Spray, 45ml	___ Hydrocortisone 1% crm, 15 gm
__ Pseudoephedrine 30mg/5ml liq., 120ml	___ Tolnaftate powder, 45gm
__ Brompheniramine/Phenylephrine soln, 120ml	___ Male Condoms

B. Controlled Substances.

1. General.

   a. Controlled substances, as used here, are defined as.

      (1) Drugs or chemicals in DEA Schedules I-V: (for example, the manufacturers label for Acetaminophen with Codeine #3(30 mg.) carries the DEA symbol for Schedule III (C-III) and will be treated as a Schedule III by Coast Guard units.). NOTE: The use of Schedule I, II, III, IV, and V is synonymous to CI, CII, CIII, CIV, and CV, respectively.

      (2) Precious metals.

      (3) Ethyl alcohol (excluding denatured).

      (4) Other drugs or materials the local CO or Pharmacy and Therapeutics Committee determine to have significant abuse potential.

   b. CG authorized uses for controlled substances are one of the following.

      (1) Medicinal purposes.

      (2) Retention as evidence in legal or disciplinary actions.

      (3) Other uses CG Regulations specifically authorize.

   c. Controlled substances not authorized.

      (1) Amphetamines for fatigue management or performance enhancement (go-pills).

      (2) Ephedra derivatives, including ephedrine.

      (3) Controlled substances for weight loss, including human chorionic gonadotropin (HCG).

      (4) Schedule I (or CI) drugs.

      (5) Alcoholic beverages.

   d. Quantity Definitions. Due to the potential for abuse and associated audits required, and the DoD Pharmaceutical Prime Vendor ordering advantage, CG regional practice site pharmacies should strive to maintain minimal quantities of controlled substances based solely on the prescribing habits of its providers.

2. Custody and Controlled Substance Audits.

   a. Controlled Substance Custodian (CSC).

      (1) Pharmacy Officers, when assigned, shall be appointed in writing as the CSC by the Regional Practice Manager (RPM).

      (2) In the absence of a Pharmacy Officer, RPM shall designate the Health Services Administrator (HSA) as the CSC.

      (3) Medical and Dental Officers may not serve as alternate CSCs, which avoids a possible conflict of interest.

(4) Temporarily assigned personnel shall not serve as CSCs or alternates.

(5) Under United States Coast Guard Regulations 1992, COMDTINST M5000.3 (series), Chapter 6-2-3-A-(6), the XO is directly responsible for medical matters if a Medical Officer is not assigned. For sickbays, the CO shall designate a commissioned officer as the CSC.

(6) An inventory audit of all controlled substances is required whenever the CSC is changed. Documentation of this type of audit will be forwarded, signed and retained as every controlled substance audit (Chapter 10-B-2-b-1-b). At the time of this change in designation and subsequent inventory audit, all keys should be transferred and/or combination locks changed.

b. Unit Controlled Substance Audits.

(1) Controlled Substance Audit Boards (CSAB). Each regional practice site pharmacy procuring, storing, or dispensing controlled substances shall have a CSAB.

(a) Membership: The CSAB shall consist of two or more disinterested members, E-6 or above, designated in writing by the RPM. CSAB letters of designation will remain in effect until the members are relieved in writing or detached from the command. In no case may the controlled substance custodian be a member of the CSAB. A DISINTERESTED MEMBER is defined as one not assigned or directly involved in daily regional practice site operations.

(b) The CSAB shall conduct monthly audits of controlled substances at regional practice sites (quarterly on afloat sickbays) and submit the report to the RPM for signature within 5 working days. The RPM will review the report, sign it, make a copy for their records upload the report to the CG Portal Microsite and then forward the signed original CSAB report to the pharmacy for retention. The regional practice site pharmacy will retain for three (3) years.

(c) Monthly, CSABs shall audit all working and bulk stock of C-II through C-V controlled substances, precious metals, ethyl alcohol, and drugs or other items locally designated as controlled substances due to abuse potential and report all quantities on Monthly Report for Narcotics and Other Controlled Drugs, Form CG-5353 or CHCS generated controlled substance vault report.

(d) During monthly audits, CSABs shall inspect controlled substances for expiration, deterioration, and inadequate or improper labeling. Expired products or those with other discrepancies shall be removed for disposal.

(e) The CSAB shall count the required controlled substances, review a representative random sample of prescriptions, receipts and issue documents, and report the results on Monthly Report for Narcotics and Other Controlled Drugs, Form CG-5353 or the CHCS generated controlled substance vault report form. For sealed containers, a bottle count is sufficient; for open containers an exact count is required. For open liquid containers, an estimate other than an exact volume measurement is adequate. CSABs may use tamper-proof seals on open containers to avoid future counting of partial quantities.

(f) CSAB members shall be advised that the CG health care program is committed to the privacy of patient health information. Federal laws (the Privacy Act and the Health Insurance Portability and Accountability Act [HIPAA]) govern uses and disclosures of medical information.

(g) During the CSAB process, respect patient privacy: do not access information you do not need for CSAB tasks, do not discuss patient information with anyone outside the CSAB. HIPAA is Federal law and violations may mean civil penalties up to $50,000 and/or criminal penalties. It is to be reminded that these laws also govern how ones information is protected while even a patient in any CG/DoD health care facility.

(2) DEA Biennial Inventories. To comply with DEA requirements, all controlled substances shall be inventoried by the custodian during <u>May of even-numbered</u> years. This copy of the Monthly/Quarterly Report for Narcotics and Other Controlled Drugs, Form CG-5353 or CHCS generated controlled substance vault report shall be maintained on file locally in the pharmacy and will be labeled "FOR DEA BIENNIAL INVENTORY" at the top of the form.

3. <u>Drug Enforcement Administration (DEA) Registration</u>.

a. DEA registration is required for those CG regional practice site pharmacies with Prime Vender (PV) ordering capability. Purchase of controlled substances from commercial sources is prohibited unless approved and procured by the Regional Pharmacy Executive (RPE) of the practice site. Sickbays shall not register with the DEA unless in-house physician services are provided. The regional practice site's Drug Enforcement Agency Registration, Form DEA-244A, shall be forwarded to the HSWL SC Pharmacy Officer as the approving authority for "fee exempt" status for processing of the regional practice site DEA certificates.

b. The HSWL SC shall forward the Drug Enforcement Agency Registration, Form DEA-244A to the DEA, providing a copy to the originating regional practice site pharmacy. The DEA will issue the registration directly to the practice site.

c. In the case of DEA renewals, (FACILITY RENEWALS ONLY--NOT INDIVIDUAL PROVIDERS), do not complete. Send the entire renewal application to the HSWL SC Pharmacy Officer via traceable means (e.g. DHS authorized Commercial Carriers FedEx or UPS), who will electronically complete and submit the renewal application. For questions regarding renewal of clinic DEA certificates, contact the HSWL SC Pharmacy Officer for further guidance.

4. Reporting Theft or Loss. Theft or loss of controlled substance is defined as any discrepancy for which all accountability process has been exhausted with negative results. NOTE: Overage or shortage of one (1) to two (2) tablets/capsules from a newly opened bottle of controlled substance does not constitute theft or loss but shall be notated in the Perpetual Inventory as manufacturer's bottling discrepancy. Immediately, upon discovery of ANY discrepancy the HSWL SC Pharmacy Officer will be notified for guidance.

   a. If discovered during the course of a monthly CSAB, a designated command member shall contact the HSWL SC Pharmacy Officer, discuss the circumstances of the discrepancy, and request guidance for further action. The HSWL SC Pharmacy Officer will advise the RPM and SHSO in writing or by e-mail of the guidance provided. Should the HSWL SC Pharmacy Officer determine an investigation is warranted, the HSWL SC Commanding Officer (CO) shall appoint one or more members to investigate the discrepancy. The HSWL SC CO shall not appoint CSAB members or interested members to investigate an incident they have reported.

   b. If discovered other than during the course of a monthly CSAB, the CSC, via the regional practice site's proper chain of command, shall notify the HSWL SC Pharmacy Officer and request guidance for further action. Guidelines as indicated in Chapter 10-B-4-a. may be followed, if warranted.

      (1) Finding of the investigational review shall be forwarded to the HSWL SC Pharmacy Officer.

      (2) The HSWL SC Pharmacy Officer shall determine if the discrepancy warrants further action or DEA notification via Report of Theft or Loss of Controlled Substances, Form DEA-106. A copy of all Report of Theft or Loss of Controlled Substances, Form DEA-106 reports submitted to DEA shall be sent to Commandant (CG-11).

5. Procuring, Storing, Transferring, and Disposing of Controlled Substances.

   a. Procurement.

      (1) Regional practice site pharmacies shall procure controlled substances from the DLA prime vendor source. CG vessels shall obtain authorized controlled substances through their respective RPE.

      (2) Schedule I controlled substances and alcoholic beverages are prohibited and shall not be procured or stocked in CG health care facilities

      (3) Upon receipt, controlled substances shall immediately be placed in the custody of the designated CSC. The invoice shall be reviewed and compared against the requisition, verifying receipt of all products and quantities listed on the invoice. The CSC shall acknowledge receipt by

signing and dating the invoice. Controlled substance procurement documents shall be maintained in the pharmacy for three (3) years.

b. Storage.

(1) Controlled substances shall be stored in an all-purpose GSA Class V safe. Chapter 11 of the Physical Security and Force Protection Manual, COMDTINST M5530.1 (series), offers in-depth guidance regarding storage of Controlled Substances.

(2) For CANA (Diazepam 10mg Auto Injectors) acquisition and storage, required quantities are often too bulky to feasibly store in Class V safes. Therefore, storage in a secured locked cabinet in a controlled access and temperature controlled area is authorized. For field deployments, CANA is authorized to be stored in a secured portable container under the control and custody of the unit's CO or the designated CSC in a controlled access area. CANA must be stored between 59-86 degrees F. If this temperature cannot be maintained, a log must be maintained, indicating storage temperature and conditions with regular readings entered. Disposition of CANA shall be documented on the Perpetual Inventory of Narcotics, Alcohol, and Controlled Drugs, Form NAVMED 6710/5, from time of receipt to issuance to the primary user. For field deployments, an issue log signed by the recipient is an acceptable form of documentation. Transfer of CANA between units shall be documented via Requisition and Invoice/Shipping Document, Form DD-1149. Regional practice site pharmacies and sickbays are required to include CANA as a part of its Controlled Substance Audits.

(3) Afloat units may use existing "built in" containers to store controlled substances. Such "built in" units shall be secured at all times with positive control.

c. Transfer.

(1) Controlled substances may be transferred between CG and other government facilities using the Requisition and Invoice/Shipping Document, Form DD-1149. When completed, the document shall include.

(a) Names of issuing and receiving facility or unit.

(b) Name, strength, and quantity of each drug.

(c) Date.

(d) Signatures of the issuing and receiving custodians.

(2) Both units shall adjust inventories as required and file copies of the Requisition and Invoice/Shipping Document, Form DD-1149 for three (3) years.

(3) When the transaction cannot be completed face-to-face, documentation will be completed and then send the entire renewal application to the HSWL SC Pharmacy Officer via traceable means (e.g. DHS authorized

Commercial Carriers FedEx or UPS). The shipment document shall be maintained by the issuing unit until a signed copy of the Requisition and Invoice/Shipping Document, Form DD-1149, is returned.

(4) A copy of the Requisition and Invoice/Shipping Document, Form DD-1149, shall be sent to the regional practice site's RPE.

d. Disposal.

(1) Expired, contaminated, excessive, inadequately labeled, damaged or otherwise unusable controlled substances shall be properly labeled, isolated in the Controlled Substance Safe from usable and in-date items and included in the next shipment of pharmaceutical returns goods for credit or destruction. Pharmacy personnel will acquire a signed and dated inventory summary from the returns goods vendor prior to the transfer of returned controlled substances.

6. Prescribing Practices.

a. Authorized (Active Duty) prescribers (see Chapter 10-A-2-a). are exempt from registration under provision of 21 CFR 1301.25. The officer's social security number may be used in lieu of a DEA or NPI registration number when prescribing medications dispensed at the regional practice site pharmacy. This exemption does not apply when the officer prescribes controlled substances outside of his or her official duties. In that case, the prescriber is required to register with the DEA, at his or her own expense, and comply with applicable state and federal laws.

b. Signatures

(1) All prescriptions for controlled substances shall be signed by a medical or dental provider. For medical provider prescriptions generated in PGUI or by POE and signed electronically in the CHCS system, the pharmacy staff will generate a duplicate pharmacy label of the ordered controlled substance, placing it on a prescription blank and the patient will sign and date the back of the prescription as designated in Chapter 10-B-6-b-(4). If no medical or dental provider is assigned at the regional practice site/sickbay, the prescription shall be signed by the senior health services department representative and countersigned by the XO.

(2) All schedule II controlled substance prescriptions written by midlevel providers (i.e. Physician Assistants or Nurse Practitioners) shall be countersigned quarterly by their supervising Medical Officer.

(3) The back of all controlled substance prescriptions shall include the wording "RECEIVED BY:" followed by the patient's signature, address, the date dispensed, and quantity received by the patient. Recommended is made that the patient observe the amount dispensed during the course of the second (dual integrity) count or at time of dispensing.

c. Quantities and Refills.

(1) Controlled substances shall be prescribed in minimal quantities consistent with proper treatment of the patient's condition. Controlled substance prescriptions generated from a source other than the CG regional practice site may only be honored for formulary items at the practice site where a registered pharmacist is available and at the discretion of the pharmacist.

(2) Out-of-state controlled substance prescriptions may be dispensed if, in the professional judgment of the RPE, the prescription appears legitimate. These prescriptions should invoke special scrutiny by the RPE/registered pharmacist.

(3) Schedule II prescriptions shall not be accepted more than seven days after the date the prescription was written. For Schedule III through V, prescriptions will not be accepted more than 30 days after the date the prescription was written.

(4) Schedule II prescriptions shall be limited to a maximum of 30 day supply. The only exception shall be medication for Attention Deficit Disorder (ADD) where quantities may be dispensed in up to a 90 day supply. Refills are not permitted on Schedule II drugs.

(5) Schedule III, IV, and V prescriptions shall be limited to 30-day quantities with up to five refills within a 180 day period and only when authorized by the prescriber. The only exception shall be for chronic seizure medications, which may be dispensed in up to 90-day quantities with one refill (six months' total supply). Prescriptions generated at sources outside of a CG regional practice facility shall only be honored for these quantities, at the discretion of the pharmacist. Patients shall be informed of this quantity or refill limitation at the time of the initial prescription presentation, allowing the patient the opportunity to have the prescription(s) filled elsewhere.

(6) Controlled prescriptions shall not be commonly filled until the patient, for whom it is intended, is available to pick up the medication. This should also include refills. However, if a pharmacy's workload is such that in the opinion of the Pharmacist it is in the best interest to maintain pharmacy flow, refill of controlled substances may be completed in advance as long as the pharmacy personnel ensures positive and secured control until the patient picks up the medication. These refills shall be bagged and/or sealed in such a way to ensure tamper resistance. Additionally, they shall be housed in a central location such that at the end of the day, those controlled prescriptions not picked up shall be returned to the narcotics safe for storage.

d. Filing Prescriptions.

(1) Controlled substance prescriptions shall be serially numbered and maintained in two files:

(2) File #1: All C-II, precious metals, and alcohol prescriptions.

(3) File #2: All C-III, C-IV, and C-V prescriptions.

(4) All prescriptions shall be maintained on file for three (3) years after which they may be destroyed by shredding.

(5) All controlled prescriptions shall be posted on Perpetual Inventory of Narcotics, Alcohol, and Controlled Drugs, Form NAVMED 6710/5 at the time of each transaction. A physical back count of the opened container from which the prescription was dispensed will be conducted to verify the remaining balance. The prescription shall then be diagonally lined across and initialed by the pharmacy staff member completing the transaction.

C. Forms and Records.

1. General. Records shall be maintained for certain procedures conducted within all CG regional practice site locations. Among mandatory requirements for record keeping are the prescribing of drugs, handling of controlled substances, and quality control procedures. Standardized forms are available for all procedures except quality control.

2. Prescription Forms.

   a. Regional practice site providers shall write prescriptions on the DoD Prescription blank, Form DD-1289 or equivalent, when chart prescribing, PGUI or POE is not available.

   b. All prescriptions shall be filed in one of three files:

      (1) All non-controlled drug prescriptions;

      (2) Schedule II prescriptions; and,

      (3) Schedule III, IV, and V prescriptions.

   c. Prescriptions will be written in black or blue ink, indelible pencil, or typewritten must show the information:

      (1) Patient's full name.

      (2) Date the prescription was written.

      (3) Full generic name (or trade name with substitution instructions), dosage form desired, and dosage size or strength written in the metric system. The quantity dispensed shall be clearly specified numerically ("one bottle" or "one package" are not acceptable). When controlled prescriptions are written, the numeric quantity shall also be written out and in parentheses next to the numeric amount (e.g. Disp. 12 (twelve) tablets). Standard pharmacy abbreviations may be used in writing dispensing and dosage instructions but not in specifying the drug to be dispensed.

      (4) Complete, explicit and distinct directions to the patient are required on all prescriptions. Expressions such as "take as directed," "label," etc. are NOT allowed.

      (5) Prescriber's legible, legal signature (initials not permitted) with printed or stamped name and professional discipline (MD, DO, DMD, DDS, PA, HS2, etc.). When CG provider order entry or PGUI entry is utilized, electronic signature satisfies this requirement

      (6) All additional requirements when prescribing controlled substances:

         (a) Patients complete address.

         (b) Prescriber's SSN, DEA or NPI number.

         (c) NOTE: Alterations on prescriptions for CII controlled substances are prohibited.

d. Multiple prescription forms, such as Poly Prescription, Form NAVMED 6710/6 or Prescription Limited, Poly, Form NAVMED 6710/10, which are intended for use when prescribing a number of non-controlled drugs for one patient, are authorized.

e. Maintenance of all prescriptions on file, including all "prescription logs" related to chart prescribing is required for three (3) years, after which they may be destroyed by shredding.

f. The pharmacy shall have readily retrievable access to the patient's medical information, including provider's current patient visit entry, patient's current medications, age, allergies, weight, etc., when preparing and dispensing prescriptions.

3. Quality Control Forms. Quality control is important for proper conformity and safety of drug products to be dispensed. The two main areas that benefit from quality control are compounding and prepackaging. A locally prepared form shall be used, which provides clearly definable material sources (manufacturer's name, lot numbers, and expiration dates), procedures used, intermediary and final checks by supervisory personnel, and labeling.

4. Controlled Drug Forms.

a. Narcotic and Controlled Drug Inventory-24 Hours, Form NAVMED 6710/4. This record shall be maintained at CG regional practice site locations, providing inpatient care.

(1) The Narcotic and Controlled Drug Inventory-24 Hours, Form NAVMED 6710/4 shall be signed by the senior health services technician on each watch after the drugs have been checked prior to relief. The drugs shall be checked concurrently by the HS reporting for duty as well as by the HS being relieved. Any discrepancies noted shall be reported immediately. The record is used for two (2) weeks, with a one (1) week period on each side. The night HS shall initiate the record.

(2) The serial numbers of new Narcotic and Controlled Drug Account Record, Form NAVMED 6710/1 received from the pharmacy during each watch shall be entered. The serial numbers of completed Narcotic and Controlled Drug Account Record, Form NAVMED 6710/1 returned to the pharmacy shall be entered and the Pharmacist or authorized representative shall acknowledge receipt by initialing in the appropriate column.

(3) At the time specified in local instructions, the senior health services technician shall audit the clinic controlled substances supplies. After the audit, the senior health services technician shall date and sign the Narcotic and Controlled Drug Inventory-24 Hours, Form NAVMED 6710/4.

b. Narcotic and Controlled Drug Account Record, Form NAVMED 6710/1.

(1) Upon receipt of a properly completed prescription requisition, a separate Narcotic and Controlled Drug Account Record, Form NAVMED 6710/1

shall be prepared by the pharmacy for each Schedule II through Schedule V drug, and any other drug which requires control procedures.

(2) All Narcotic and Controlled Drug Account Records, Form NAVMED 6710/1 shall be kept in a controlled drug book.

(3) All entries shall be made in blue or black ink. Errors shall be corrected by drawing a single line through the erroneous entry and having the person making the correction sign the entry. The correct entry shall be recorded on the following line, if necessary.

(4) If a new issue is received before the old issue is completely expended, the new Narcotic and Controlled Drug Account Record, Form NAVMED 6710/1 shall be inserted in back of the current record. The serial number of the new Narcotic and Controlled Drug Account Record, Form NAVMED 6710/1 shall be entered on the Narcotic and Controlled Drug Inventory-24 Hours, Form NAVMED 6710/4.

(5) The heading for each Narcotic and Controlled Drug Account Record, Form NAVMED 6710/1 shall be completed at the time of issue. The body shall be used for recording expenditures and balances only.

(6) Each time a drug is used, complete information shall be recorded: date, time, patient, prescriber's name, dispenser, amount used, and balance remaining on hand on the Narcotic and Controlled Drug Account Record, Form NAVMED 6710/1.

   (a) All amounts will be recorded in Arabic numerals. If the unit of measure is a milliliter (ml) and the amount used is less than one ml, it shall be recorded as a decimal (e.g., 0.5 ml) rather than a fraction.

   (b) When a fraction of the amount is expended to the patient, it shall be placed in parentheses before the amount recorded in the expended column; [e.g., an entry of (0.0005)1 on the morphine sulfate 16 mg/ml record indicates that one-half ml was expended and that 0.008 gm was administered].

   (c) If a single dose of a controlled substance is accidentally damaged or contaminated during preparation for administration or the patient refuses after preparation, the dose shall be destroyed and a brief statement of the circumstances shall be entered on the Narcotic and Controlled Drug Account Record, Form NAVMED 6710/1. Such statements shall be signed and witnessed by two (2) health service providers.

   (d) If multiple doses of a controlled substance are damaged, another senior HS shall record the disposition of the drug, including date, amount of drug, brief statement of disposition, and new balance. Both the senior and witnessing HS shall sign the Narcotic and Controlled Drug Account Record, Form NAVMED 6710/1.

   (e) Deteriorated drugs shall be returned to the pharmacy for disposal.

(f) The completed Narcotic and Controlled Drug Account Record, Form NAVMED 6710/1, along with the counter-type dispenser, shall be returned to the pharmacy.

(g) Monthly, the pharmacy shall report all Narcotic and Controlled Drug Account Records, Form NAVMED 6710/1 still outstanding 30 days from date of issue. The report shall be verified and returned to the pharmacy for reconciliation. Discrepancies shall be reported to the RPE via the Controlled Substances Audit Board Inventory Report.

c. Narcotic and Controlled Drug Book

(1) Each activity drawing controlled substances from the pharmacy shall maintain a loose leaf notebook containing Narcotic and Controlled Drug Inventory-24 Hours, Form NAVMED 6710/4 in the first section and individual Narcotic and Controlled Drug Account Record, Form NAVMED 6710/1 in the latter sections.

(2) The senior HS shall remove all filled Narcotic and Controlled Drug Inventory-24 Hours, Form NAVMED 6710/4 over three (3) months old from the Narcotic and Controlled Drug Book and return them to the pharmacy.

d. Perpetual Inventory of Narcotics, Alcohol, and Controlled Drugs, Form NAVMED 6710/5. Separate Perpetual Inventory of Narcotics, Alcohol, and Controlled Drugs, Form NAVMED 6710/5 forms are not required for each controlled substance (C-II through C-V) when electronic records or documentation are available via the Composite Health Care System (CHCS) or equivalent software programs. The requirement for hard copy monthly substance audit board report, Monthly Report For Narcotics and Other Controlled Drugs, Form CG-5353 is still required, however, the CHCS software prepares and automates controlled substance inventory reports which are acceptable and can be used as an equivalent to the Monthly Report For Narcotics And Other Controlled Drugs, Form CG-5353. If software is not consistently available, prepare a separate Perpetual Inventory of Narcotics, Alcohol, and Controlled Drugs, Form NAVMED 6710/5 for each controlled substance (C-II through C-V). All boxes and columns below are self-explanatory except as noted:

(1) Drug Name. Enter generic or proprietary drug name as appropriate, e.g., "Codeine Sulfate.

(2) Strength. Express as gm, mg, etc.

(3) Unit. Enter dosage form as appropriate.

(4) Prescription or Requisition Number. Enter appropriate prescription or requisition (voucher) number. For issues returned to the pharmacy, the source will be entered.

(5) Recipient. Enter "pharmacy" for receipts. Enter regional practice site or patient name, as appropriate, for expenditures.

(6) Narcotic and Controlled Drug Account Records, Form NAVMED 6710/1 Returned. The date the Narcotic and Controlled Drug Account Records, Form NAVMED 6710/1 is returned to the pharmacy shall be entered on the appropriate line bearing the same serial number or prescription number.

5. Forms Availability.

a. Obtain DEA forms from the nearest DEA office. Consult with the regional practice site's RPE for more information.

b. Prescription Blanks. Prescription blanks DoD Prescription, Form DD-1289 can be found at the following web site:
http://www.dtic.mil/whs/directives/infomgt/forms/formsprogram.htm

D. Drug Dispensing Without a Medical Officer.

 1. General. Health Services Technicians (HSs) dispensing prescriptions without a Medical Officer's direct supervision, (e.g., at independent duty shore stations or vessels), shall be conducted in accordance with provisions of this manual and the Health Services Allowance List. These services shall be provided for active duty personnel only. HSs in these situations are encouraged to seek consultation with their Regional Pharmacy Executive (RPE).

 2. Child-Resistant Containers. Prepackaged OTC products shall be issued in their original container. For vessels, limited quantities of prescription drugs may be issued in labeled plastic zip-lock bags and retained by the patient while underway with proper labeling including name of patient, name of medication, exact instructions, precautions, and warnings regarding the medication, date dispensed, and initials of dispenser. However, these bags must be inserted in a child resistant container with proper labeling when removed from the vessel.

 3. Controlled Substances.

    a. All drugs shall be dispensed under the supervision of a Health Services Technician at activities where there are no officers of the health services department.

    b. An officer (usually the XO), designated by the CO, shall serve as the Controlled Substance Custodian (CSC) and keep in a separate locked compartment, all bulk un-issued controlled substances, alcohol, or items otherwise controlled. The CSC shall always maintain positive control of the keys or combination. The CSC shall arrange for the care and safe custody of all keys and require strict compliance with instructions concerning the receipt, custody, and issue of controlled substances and alcohol as contained in the law, Coast Guard Regulations, COMDTINST M5000.3 (series) and this Manual.

    c. The CSC or the designated Sickbay/Medical personnel shall retain the keys or combination to the working stock storage area while on duty. When relieved, they shall deliver the keys to their relief or to a responsible person designated by local instructions. A copy of the combination of a safe, if used, shall be sealed in an envelope and deposited with the CO.

    d. COs may authorize temporary deviations from the controls established in this Chapter due to operational and/or emergency situations.

    e. Controlled Substance Audit Board (CSAB) at these units (e.g., Cutters) shall be conducted at least quarterly by two disinterested members. CSAB shall also be conducted when there is a change in designation of the CSC and when there is a permanent change in Sickbay/Medical personnel. Chapter 10.B. provides detailed instructions regarding CSAB.

4. <u>Formulary</u>. Health Services Technicians on independent duty corpsmen (IDHS) shall maintain drug formularies consisting of:

   a. Standardized Health Services Drug Formulary items.

   b. Health Services Allowance List Afloat requirements.

   c. Chronic medications prescribed by a physician for active duty members currently assigned to the duty station.

   d. Other drugs the HS has been authorized in writing by the DMOA to stock for their active duty members. A copy of the DMOA's written approval of these medications will be forwarded to the RPE for review, approval and acquisition. The review will ensure compliance with the DoD Basic Core Formulary.

5. <u>Non-Prescription Medication Programs</u>. Sickbays are encouraged to operate a non-prescription medication program as described in Chapter 10-A-6-j of this Manual. HSs shall contact their RPE for guidance and additional support.

CHAPTER 11

HEALTH CARE PROCUREMENT

Section A. Contracting For Health Care Services.

Section B. Health Care Services Invoice Review and Auditing.

Section C. Claims Processing.

CHAPTER ELEVEN – HEALTH CARE PROCUREMENT

A. Contracting For Health Care Services.

1. General. Commandant (CG-11) has fiscal responsibility for health care for all CG beneficiaries. The necessary care can be obtained through contracts with private concerns and individuals and interagency and other agreements with military facilities. COs are responsible for obtaining the necessary services for each fiscal year, subject to HSWL SC review and approval. HSWL SC first authorizes all non-emergency, non-Federal health care. The HSWL SC is responsible for all health services contracting in its area and shall comply with Federal Acquisition Regulations Part 37. The HSWL SC oversees all non-Federal care acquired and minimizes expenses by ensuring competitive contracting procedures take place.

2. Type of Services. The following services may be procured by contract as determined by the HSWL SC.

   a. Allergist.

   b. Dental Prosthetic Laboratory.

   c. Dentist, Dental Hygienist, or chairside Dental Assistant.

   d. General Medicine (Physician or Midlevel Providers).

   e. Group Practice Hospital.

   f. Gynecologist.

   g. Medical Laboratory.

   h. Neurologist.

   i. Nurse (Registered or Licensed Practical).

   j. Obstetrician.

   k. Occupational Health Services (for OCCMED Physicals).

   l. Optometrist.

   m. Orthopedist.

   n. Pharmacist.

   o. Physical Therapist or Certified Athletic Trainer.

   p. Psychiatrist or Psychologist.

q. Radiologist.

3. <u>Eligibility For Contract Health Care Services</u>. Eligibility for contract health care services is the same as described in Chapter 2.

    a. The following persons are NOT eligible for health care services rendered by contract providers:

        (1) Family members of CG personnel and retired and retired members of the CG (however, they may receive health care services when the contractor performs the service at a CG Clinic or sickbay and/or if the CG has contracted with a health care provider as a demonstration project).

        (2) Active duty beneficiaries separated from the Service while undergoing treatment (eligibility for treatment terminates and becomes the member's responsibility).

        (3) CG civilian employees except for required Occupational Medical Surveillance and Evaluation Program (OMSEP) physical examinations and required pre-appointment examinations, all funded using HSWL SC funds.

    b. Dental laboratory fees for non-active duty beneficiaries:

        (1) <u>Retirees</u>. Retirees are authorized to use private sector dental laboratories. Pay retirees' dental laboratory fees in the same manner as for active duty members.

        (2) <u>Dependents</u>. The dependent receiving the treatment shall pay all private sector laboratory fees resulting from space-available treatment . A suggested way to handle such payments is to require dependents to submit a check or money order payable to the private sector laboratory before delivery of appliances. The attending Dental Officer then photocopies the check or money order, pays the laboratory, and retains the photocopy in the dental record.

4. <u>Approval to Contract for Services</u>.

    a. Units shall submit letter requests for contract health care services through the appropriate chain of command to the HSWL SC. All requests must contain this information:

        (1) Description of services required (e.g., general health care, pharmacy, lab, or specialty care such as OB/GYN, optometry, or psychiatry), including desired days and hours of availability.

        (2) A justification of the need for the service.

(3) Estimated annual cost of the required services.

(4) A list of USMTFs within 40 miles of the unit and whether they could perform the desired service.

(5) A list of CG units benefiting from the services.

(6) The number of active duty members assigned to each unit.

(7) Either the names and mailing addresses of all interested, recommended providers or a justification of other than full, open competition (see Chapter 11-A-7, Pre-contract Award Actions, below).

(8) Preferred solicitation area and the rationale for it (e.g. "provider must be located within 20 miles of the unit", etc.).

(9) Estimated number of annual CG visits to the provider.

(10) A list (by type) of any other approved or requested health care contracts.

b. Each request must be able to stand on its own merits and fulfill cost-to-benefit criteria. HSWL SC will analyze each request and provide written approval or disapproval (with alternative proposals) to the requesting unit through the chain of command. If approved, the HSWL SC Contracting Officer will undertake procurement.

c. HSWL SC will not renew existing contracts simply as a matter of convenience. Each contract must continue to prove its value annually on a cost-to-benefit basis before its renewal. HSWL SC will review each contract's current fiscal year activity. If the contract passes review, it may be renewed; if it does not, HSWL SC will so advise the unit receiving the contract services.

5. <u>Funding</u>.

a. The HSWL SC shall budget, review, and pay for all HSWL SC authorized non-Federal health care obtained in its area. These documents contain detailed instructions:

(1) HSWL SC Standing Operating Procedures (HSWL SC SOP), Annex D.

(2) HSWL SC Instruction M6000.1 (series).

b. Charge all HSWL SC authorized non-Federal health care expenditures to the HSWL SC AFC-57 account. HSWL SC can find detailed object class and cost center information in the Accounting Manual, COMDTINST M7300.4 (series).

6. <u>Pre-contract Award Actions</u>.

    a.   The Contracting Officer issues solicitations to obtain supplies and services from industry on a competitive (more than 1 source) or non-competitive (1 source) basis. The Competition in Contracting Act of 1984, (PL-98-369) requires the Government to contract for supplies and services by means of full, open competition to the maximum extent possible. This means all responsible firms or individuals who can provide the supplies or services must be allowed to compete for a government contract. Contracting Officers locate potential contractors by publishing the proposed procurement in the Commerce Business Daily as required by Federal Acquisition Regulation (FAR), Part 5.

        (1) <u>Non-competitive Procurements</u>. Pre-awarding a firm a Government contract violates the Competition in Contracting Act of 1984. If it is claimed only one firm can provide the supplies or service, the purchasing office must justify in writing other than full, open competition, setting forth the facts and rationale (see FAR, Part 6) to support this claim. The justification must be certified that it is accurate and complete and send it with the purchase request when sending it to the contracting officer for procurement action.

        (2) <u>Competitive Procurements</u>. The Contracting Officer also may require certain information before contracting on a competitive basis. The Contracting Officer may request the types of information below to determinate responsibility within the meaning of Federal Acquisition Regulation, Part 9.

            (a) Organizational structure and plan to accomplish the service.

            (b) Summary of experience in performing the same or similar work.

            (c) Evidence of pertinent state and local licenses.

            (d) Evidence of professional liability insurance, or that the offeror can obtain such insurance.

            (e) Membership in professional organizations.

            (f) Resume of key personnel with particular emphasis on academic achievements pertinent to the proposed services.

            (g) Information about the firm or its key individuals that reflects their status or professional recognition in their field, e.g., awards, published articles, and the like.

    b.   <u>Pre-award survey</u>. Subject to the Contracting Officer's approval, a visit may be made to the offeror's facility before the award (pre-award survey) to review some of the above data to reduce submitted data. The following paragraphs are examples of the information that may be required from an offer or

(1) Brief description of the facility, how long established, where located relative to the required mile radius, daily operating hours, weekly operating hours (include holidays, Saturdays, and Sundays).

(2) Brief description of similar work performed under Government contracts including the government agency's name, contract number, contract price, and name and telephone number of the agency's contracting officer.

(3) A resume, X pages maximum, including education, past and present experience over the last X years, certificates, association membership, etc., of the key persons who will perform the work under the contract and their letter of intent indicating they intend to work for the offeror if it is awarded the medical services contract.

c. Qualifications. Minimum qualifications required to perform the contract may be stated; however, these qualification requirements must be justified. For example:

(1) Personnel.

 (a) Physician. At a minimum, a X year degree in medicine from an accredited college, license to practice medicine in the location where the services will be performed, member of the AMA; X years' experience in practicing general medicine.

 (b) Nurse. RN or LPN. B.S. degree (or equivalent) in nursing from an accredited college; ANA-certified or equivalent; X years' experience in handling patients, administering patient records, etc.

 (c) Laboratory Technician. HHS certified, ASCP or eligible, X years' experience in all phases of laboratory work; e.g., x-rays, blood samples, etc.

(2) Facility.

 (a) Within a X mile radius of the CG facility requiring the services.

 (b) Capable of accommodating or rendering services for at least X patients simultaneously.

7. Award Evaluation Factors.

    a. State the steps or procedures to be used to evaluate the proposals.

    b. List the evaluation criteria in the descending order of relative importance and state whether one factor will have predominant consideration over another. For example:

        (1) Personnel.

        (2) Experience.

        (3) Facility.

        (4) Price.

    c. Establish the criteria to be used in evaluating the proposal. They must be the same as the evaluation factors for award the solicitation cited. The weights assigned to the factors may be in any form, e.g., adjective (acceptable, outstanding), numerical (50). Give this information to the Contracting Officer, preferably before he or she issues the solicitation, but in any event before receiving the proposals for evaluation.

8. Post-Contract Award Actions.

    a. Referring for Contract Services. Before referring any person to a medical services contractor, the cognizant authority shall determine whether:

        (1) The person is eligible.

        (2) Services are available in-house.

        (3) Services are available from a USMTF.

        (4) Services are available from another Federal facility, e.g., Department of Veterans Affairs, under an interagency support agreement.

    b. Contracting Officer's Technical Representative. The contracting office that awarded the contract administers it. If the requiring office requests, a Contracting Officer's Technical Representative (COTR) may be assigned to the contract. The COTR is preferably a health services program manager or medical administration officer having jurisdiction in the contract services area. The Contracting Officer designates the Contracting Officer's Technical Representative in a written, signed letter of appointment describing the COTR's responsibilities and limitations. These responsibilities and limitations must strictly be adhered to avoid any conflicts with the contractor about changes to contract terms and conditions.

    c. Health Care Invoices.

        (1) Contractor Invoices.

(a) All invoices for health care services contractors by contractors shall be processed for payment under the applicable contract's terms and conditions. This Manual's Chapter 2 describes certifying and processing non-Federal health care invoices. The Contracting Officer is responsible for including the applicable invoice and payment clauses (e.g., Federal Acquisition Regulations 52.204-3, Taxpayer Identification, 52.232-25, Prompt Payment, etc.) in the contract. Ensure the contracting officer also includes these invoice requirements in the contract so the invoice is proper for payment:

   (1) An itemized, priced list of the services by contract or order line item number.

   (2) Any additional information deemed necessary to process the invoice for payment.

(b) In addition to the invoice requirements above any invoice without the following supporting documentation will not be paid.

   (1) Services Rendered Under Non-Emergent Conditions. A referral slip or written confirmation of patient's eligibility from cognizant health services department representative.

   (2) Services Rendered Under Emergent Conditions. A written statement from the patient describing the emergent condition(s). The cognizant health services department representative must certify the patient's eligibility and emergent condition.

(c) If the eligible patient pays the contractor for services rendered under a contract and requests reimbursement, the reimbursement claim must be submitted to the appropriate accounting office on Public Voucher for Purchases and Services Other Than Personal, Form SF-1034. A patient's invoice cannot be reimbursed from funds obligated under a contract even though the contractor rendered the services. These documents must accompany the claim:

   (1) The contractor's itemized invoice.

   (2) A copy of the invoice and receipt showing payment to the contractor.

   (3) The patient's written statement of the circumstances justifying the claim.

        (4) The cognizant health services department representative's approval of the claim.

  (2) Invoices outside the CONUS.

      (a) The nearest CG facility having an authorized certifying officer shall process invoices for emergency health care from civilian facilities furnish to CG members. The invoices and justification explaining the reasons for the emergency health care must be attached to the Claim for Reimbursement for Expenditures on Official Business, Form SF-1164.

      (b) Every attempt to pay for emergency health care should be made before departing from a foreign port to reduce paperwork and pay at the exchange rate. For emergency care under $2500.00 the Imprest Fund may be used. If payment prior to departure is not feasible, advise the facility rendering the service to send all invoices to the United States Embassy or appropriate consular office for the area.

Figure 11.A.1

STATEMENT OF WORK

1. Scope. Provide all labor, materials, and facilities necessary to perform the tasks herein.

2. Definitions.

   a. Patient. An eligible CG military member.

   b. Emergency. Treatment required to curtail the patient's undue suffering or loss of life or limb.

   c. Non-Elective Condition. A condition that, if untreated, would render the patient unfit for duty.

   d. Elective Procedure. Treatment the patient *desires*, e.g., vasectomy, tubal ligation, sterility test, contact lenses, orthodontics, etc.

   e. Duty Status. A determination of the patient's ability to perform the assigned tasks at the assigned work station. These statuses apply:

      (1) Fit for Full Duty (FFD). Patient is not physically restricted or limited.

      (2) Fit for Limited Duty (FLD). Patient is physically restricted or limited, e.g., office work only; no lifting, stooping, prolonged standing, walking, running, jumping, sea duty, etc.

      (3) Not Fit for Duty (NFD). Patient cannot perform any assigned tasks at assigned work station.

3. The contractor shall perform these tasks:

   a. Task I - Eligibility Determination. Provide service to the CG military personnel listed below. Each patient must show the required authorizations before the Contractor renders service.

   b. Task II - Physical Examinations. Examine the patient according to Attachment (1) requirements. [Attach copy of appropriate section of Medical Manual, COMDTINST M6000.1 (series).]

   c. Task III - Immunization. Immunize the patient and document appropriately on Immunization Record, Form SF-601 or Public Health Form 731 (International Certificate of Vaccination) in the CG Health Record the patient presents the contractor. Record also any sensitivity reactions to the immunization. The contractor shall use only those immunizing agents approved by the Department of Health and Human Services. Immunize the patient at the time intervals Attachment 2 specifies. [Attach a copy of Immunization and Chemoprophylaxis, COMDTINST M6230.4 (series).]

d. Task IV - Emergency Hospitalization. Provide all necessary services to patient while he or she is hospitalized, to a maximum of seven days. If the patient requires hospitalization for eight or more days, the contractor shall notify the CG point of contact by telephone. If the CG elects to transfer the patient to a military hospital, the contractor shall complete all necessary documents the civilian hospital may require to effect the transfer.

e. Task V - Prosthetic and Orthopedic Appliances. The contractor shall provide prosthetic or orthopedic appliances to the patient only under emergency conditions (required immediately due to his or her condition). The contractor shall document the emergency condition on the CG Health Record. Under non-emergency conditions, the contractor shall refer the patient to a military hospital to obtain these appliances.

f. Task VI - Communicable Disease. The contractor shall report all communicable diseases and recommended control measures to the CG health care provider or CO immediately after detecting the disease. The contractor also shall report to local authorities as required by local regulations.

g. Task VII - Notification. The contractor shall notify the CG health care provider or patient's CO if a patient is seriously ill, injured, or dies.

h. Task VIII - Records and Reports. For all patients the contractor shall maintain a record with this information:

(1) Outpatient Record. Record the name, rank or rating, Social Security Number, address, date of treatment, history of present illness, physical findings, diagnostic procedures including x-rays and laboratory, therapy provided, fitness for duty determination, duration and limitations if unfit or fit for limited duty, and the contractor's printed name and signature.

(2) Inpatient Report. On discharge from the hospital, furnish the patient's medical report written using diagnostic nomenclature (standard disease and operation nomenclature) to summarize the course of the case, laboratory and x-ray findings, surgeries and treatments, complications, current condition, final diagnosis, and a fitness for duty determination with duration and limitations if unfit or fit for limited duty.

Task IX - Certificate of Services. After rendering services to the patient, complete Attachment (3) and obtain the patient's signature before he or she departs from the contractor's facility or location where the services were rendered. [Attach copy of certification form.]

4. The contractor shall not execute any oral or written agreements with the patient to render a more expensive type of service than that described in the contract in which the patient pays the difference in price between the contract unit price and the price the contractor charges (for eyeglasses, see Chapter 8 Section E).

5. The contractor must obtain written authority from the patient's CG unit before filling any prescriptions.

6. The contractor must obtain written authority from the patient's CG unit before performing any elective procedure.

Personnel	Required Authorization
Active Duty	1. Valid Common Access I.D. Card 2. A referral slip signed by an authorized CG official
Reservists (Active Duty)	1. Valid Common Access I.D. Card 2. Copy of active duty orders 3. A referral slip signed by an authorized CG official
Reservists	1. Valid Common Access I.D. Card 2. A Notice of Eligibility. See Reserve Policy Manual, COMDTINST M1001.28 (series) for further details.
PHS Commissioned Officers on CG Active Duty	1. Valid Common Access I.D. Card
Prospective CG Recruit	A letter signed by an authorized official at the CG recruiting unit
The contractor shall not provide services under this contract to personnel who do not have the required authorizations listed above.	

Table 11-A-1

B. Health Care Services Invoice Review and Auditing.

    1. General.

        a. Review and audit. All health care invoices are subject to review and audit to ensure the CG pays only for necessary, appropriate health care for its beneficiaries.

            (1) The auditing process ensures the contractor's invoice charges for services provided at either reasonable fees or those in agreement with the contract.

            (2) The review process determines the appropriateness of care for the diagnosis.

        b. Discrepancies. Personnel performing the review and audit functions must remember if they find discrepancies, they must give the care provider the opportunity to comment on the findings.

        c. Conduct. The process of health care invoice auditing and review is complex and lends itself to errors; thus, most reviews and audit inquiries are not dismissed. Finding must be presented in a non-threatening manner, demonstrating the CG's willingness to cooperate with our health care providers in determining fair, equitable charges.

    2. Invoices Subject to Review and Audit. These contract and non-contract health services invoices are subject to review and audit. The unit processing the invoice should review bills in these categories before paying them:

        a. All outpatient invoices contractors submit;

        b. All inpatient and outpatient supplemental care.

    3. Review and Audit Procedures. The personnel processing health care invoices should perform these procedures:

        a. Review.

            (1) Is the diagnosis compatible with the prescribed care?

            (2) Are ancillary services (e.g., lab, x-ray, pharmacy, electrodiagnostic tests, etc.) prescribed appropriately in amount and frequency?

            (3) Is the length of care appropriate for the diagnosis?

        b. Audit. Does the contractor's invoice meet the contract definition of a proper invoice? If not, notify the Contracting Officer immediately.

            (1) Is the bill mathematically correct?

(2) Does it bill only for authorized care and services?

(3) Were services and billed care actually furnished?

(4) Do the charges agree with the provider's regular fee schedule or the prices listed in the contract?

(5) Does the bill give credit for incomplete, canceled, or partial treatments?

(6) Do dates of care match the time period the patient received the care or services?

(7) Have previous audits of this provider demonstrated billing errors?

4. <u>Report of Potential Third Party Liability, RCN 6000-2</u>. Under the Federal Medical Care Recovery Act the CG will collect the cost of health care provided to any eligible beneficiary from the appropriate insurance carrier or eligible third party. Refer to Health Care Third Party Claims Recovery, COMDTINST 6010.16 (series) for current policy. Submit this report on Report of Potential Third Party Liability, Form CG-4899.

C. Claims Processing.

1. General. The HSWL SC is responsible for processing Federal and nonfederal health care claims in compliance with the Federal Law and CG Regulations.

2. Certification. Certification ensures that only authorized payment services to eligible beneficiaries receiving health care within their entitlements and the care and related charges are appropriate. The HSWL SC shall:

   a. Administratively screen each claim and supporting documents according to Chapter 11-C-3 below. Claims submission procedures from field units are provided by the HSWL SC Standard Operating Procedures.

   b. Technically screen claims and supporting document according to Chapter 11-C-4 below. In screening, perform these actions:

      (1) Refer claims that do not satisfy the Technical Screen criteria to a medical audit staff for Appropriateness Review and/or audit.

      (2) Enter information from these claims into the Non-Federal Invoice Processing System (NIPS) data base and approve them for payment in this manner:

         (a) Claims that satisfy Administrative and Technical Screen criteria (including Active Duty Claims Program (ADCP) claims coded through a TRICARE Fiscal Intermediary).

         (b) Claims referred for Appropriateness Review and/or audit recommended for payment.

   c. Transmit payment data electronically to the CG Finance Center.

   d. Certify batch transmissions.

   e. Correct batch errors.

   f. Update vendor files.

3. Administrative Screen.

   a. Administrative screening. Administrative screening of a claim package determines the patient's authorization and eligibility to receive billed services and also ensures the package contains all appropriate, necessary documents. At a minimum, administrative screening includes:

      (1) Patient information is present and complete.

      (2) Public Voucher for Purchases and Services other than Personal, Form SF-1034 is completed for reimbursement requests.

(3) The claim is a complete, itemized original.

(4) A copy of the Report of Potential Third Party Liability, Form CG-4899 is attached if a third party is potentially liable.

(5) Verification of pre-authorization number.

(6) Support documentation is complete for Reservists' bills.

(7) Claims for formal contracts have the Contracting Officer's signature and amount to be paid.

(8) Claims for clinic support contracts have a CG beneficiary breakdown.

b. Ensure that all claims that fail to satisfy the administrative screening are corrected by the unit through the most expeditious means possible.

4. Technical Screen.

a. Health care claims must be reviewed to ensure they comply with Federal regulations. Part of that process compares claim packages to standard criteria to withstand the scrutiny of Departmental Accounting and Financial Information System (DAFIS) for payment. Technical screening of claim packages includes:

(1) Comparing charges against contract fee schedules, pre-authorizations, blanket purchase agreements, or the geographic area's usual and customary fees; claims falling within ADCP guidelines are exempt from fee review.

(2) Entering relevant claim information into NIPS.

(3) Determining whether services were appropriate for the diagnosis.

(4) Identifying claims requiring further review under these circumstances.

   (a) Unrelated charges to the initial diagnosis or injury.

   (b) Duplicate charges for services received on a given day.

   (c) Care was unauthorized or unnecessary.

   (d) Claims submitted by different providers for the same service (e.g., anesthesiology charges from more than one provider).

   (e) NIPS "flagged" the claim.

   (f) The reviewer "feels" a need for further review.

b. Claims a Technical Screen identifies for further review and/or audit require:

(1) Documentation of the problem.

(2) A recommended course of action.

5. Appropriateness Review.

    a. An Appropriateness Review is performed under these circumstances:

        (1) The HSWL SC selects or NIPS flags a claim for further review and/or audit for a Technical Screen; and/or.

        (2) Periodically for quality assurance.

    b. An Appropriateness Review requires:

        (1) An itemized claim.

        (2) A patient's signed Request for Medical Records, Form DD-877 or its' equivalent, to request medical records and other information about an individual's care. Various records, which may include.

            (a) Hospital records.

            (b) Physician's orders.

            (c) Physician and nursing progress notes.

            (d) Lab and x-ray reports.

            (e) Operative or endoscopic reports.

            (f) Admission records (history and physical examinations).

            (g) Discharge summaries.

    c. Appropriateness Review. An Appropriateness Review process often involves these activities:

        (1) Reviewing records to verify treatment of therapy was:

            (a) Appropriate for the diagnosis.

            (b) Consistent with currently accepted medical practice.

            (c) Not duplicated unnecessarily.

            (d) The length of inpatient hospitalization was appropriate for the diagnosis and course of care.

(e) The charges were reasonable; claims falling within ADCP guidelines are exempt from fee review.

(2) Obtaining additional documentation and/or correspondence from health care providers.

(3) Initially notifying health care providers of this information:

(a) Their claims are being reviewed and audited.

(b) The audit is a normal part of the CG's health care review process and does not indicate or allege the health care provider committed an offense.

(c) If reviewing cases for longer than 30 days, periodically communicate with health care providers to inform them of claim status.

d. An Appropriateness Review may recommend.

(1) Full payment for services. Enter data into and process through NIPS.

(2) Partial payment for services. Attach decision documents; recommend the amount of payment; and enter data into NIPS. Initiate a reimbursement request if the claim initially was overpaid.

(3) Consulting a specialist for peer review.

(4) Referral to a contractor for further review or an on-site hospital audit.

(5) Closing the case with no further action.

e. An Appropriateness Review includes.

(1) Fully documenting the decision process.

(2) Initiating payment or the provider's reimbursement.

(3) Drafting appropriate correspondence.

6. Peer Review.

a. A Peer Review will be performed under one of these circumstances:

(1) A health care provider objects to under these other reviews' findings.

(2) An Appropriateness Review reveals the need for a more sophisticated evaluation of the diagnosis, prognosis, or specific medical procedures employed.

b. Send the case and health care provider's additional documentation (if any) to a qualified medical, pharmaceutical, or dental specialist for review. These services should be contracted if in-house specialists are not available. Obtain a business associate agreement that the privacy, confidentiality and security of protected health information will be safeguarded in compliance with Federal and State laws.

c. Peer Review may include these detailed examinations:

   (1) Diagnosis.

   (2) Prognosis.

   (3) Appropriateness of the care provided.

   (4) Claims submitted to a Fiscal Intermediary for pricing are exempt from fee review.

   (5) Selection of the most cost-effective therapy.

d. Among other things a Pharmacist's review of pharmaceutical bills and supporting documents may include one of the following:

   (1) Determine the efficacy of prescribed medication.

   (2) Identify cost-effective choices.

   (3) Recommend stocking pharmaceuticals for future issuance.

7. Guidelines for Initial Appropriateness and Peer Reviews. These common health care services guidelines are not all-inclusive. Appropriateness and Peer Reviews should be used to assist reviewers in deciding whether in-hospital audits or contracted review services are required.

a. Trauma. Answer these questions:

   (1) Does the level of care correspond to the diagnosis?

   (2) Were appropriate facilities used?

   (3) Were laboratory and x-ray procedures appropriate? Include justification for:

      (a) Repeating procedures on a given day.

      (b) Repeating normal procedures.

      (c) Failing to follow up abnormal tests.

    (4) Were iatrogenic complications were identified appropriately? Include:

        (a) Sepsis.

        (b) Wound dehiscence.

        (c) Hemorrhage.

        (d) Pulmonary complications.

        (e) Cardiovascular complications (thrombophlebitis, etc.).

        (f) Urinary tract infection.

        (g) Anesthetic or other drug reactions (appropriate drug and dosage, known allergies).

        (h) Other associated injuries.

    (5) The length of stay was appropriate for the diagnosis and indicated complications.

    (6) The discharge diagnosis was compatible with admission diagnosis and the patient's history.

    (7) The patient's physical status on discharge:

        (a) Alive.

        (b) Complications were controlled.

        (c) Wound(s) condition was satisfactory.

        (d) Required follow-up arrangements are listed.

        (e) Medications were prescribed.

    (8) Follow-up care was appropriate, including:

        (a) Therapy.

        (b) Office visits.

        (c) Additional hospitalization was for a good reason, e.g., iatrogenic complications, continued therapy, or additional surgeries.

    (9) Fees are usual and customary for the geographic area (claims falling within ADCP guidelines are exempt from fee review).

(10) The use of multiply providers is explained.

(11) Providers' and reviewers' differences in medical opinion (particularly involving altered treatment and length of hospital stay) are significant enough to warrant negotiation.

b. <u>Laboratory Services</u>. Answer these questions:

(1) Are tests related to or necessary for the diagnosis?

(2) Were ICU standing orders in effect?

(3) Were tests repeated excessively?

(4) Were charges duplicated for the same procedure on the same day?

(5) Were tests repeated due to equipment or operator error?

(6) Were tests repeated despite normal previous test(s) (justification is required)?

(7) Were there multiple charges for the same or similar tests?

(8) Were multiple tests performed in a logical sequence (i.e., the most invasive or sophisticated performed last)?

(9) Were fees usual and customary (claims falling within ADCP guidelines are exempt from fee review)?

(10) For a laboratory under CG contract, were:

(a) Tests covered by the contract?

(b) Charges within fee schedule?

c. <u>Radiology Services</u>. Considerations:

(1) Was the examination required given the diagnosis?

(2) Were charges for portable radiology of an ambulatory patient?

(3) Were examinations repeated?

(4) Were bilateral x-rays appropriate (patients over 12 years of age)?

(5) Were charges or exams of the same anatomical part duplicated?

(6) Do examinations and in-patient dates coincide?

(7) Were examinations repeated despite normal findings in previous examinations?

d. Physical Therapy. Considerations:

(1) Was the injury or diagnosis properly documented? Did it include:

(a) Objective findings?

(b) Functional findings?

(c) Multiple provider discrepancies?

(d) Documentation of improvement?

(2) Did a physician prescribe treatment?

(3) Were injury management and treatments reasonable and necessary? Did they cover these:

(a) Was the treatment plan documented?

(b) Did objective findings permit the therapist and/or physician to monitor treatment results?

(c) Were changes in the treatment program due to unsuccessful results?

(d) Was treatment only for subjective complaints?

(e) Was the treatment related to diagnosis?

(f) Did the treatment follow standard procedures and protocols?

(g) Did the treatment plan include goals and objectives?

(4) Was the length or number of treatments excessive?

(5) Was treatment consistent or continuous or did patient attend sporadically?

(6) Did therapy continue after "Fit-For-Duty" status?

(7) Did therapy charges continue during stays in cardiac or intensive care units.

(8) Were charges duplicated for same-day, apparently inappropriate treatments?

(9) Was therapy frequency within accepted standards?

(10) Were same-day charges for three or more modalities during a single therapy session?

(11) Were charges usual and customary (claims falling within ADCP guidelines are exempt from fee review).

e. Dentistry.

    (1) For provider contract care, were:

        (a) Services within the contract scope?

        (b) Charges within fee schedules?

    (2) For emergency care, were:

        (a) Services within the scope of entitlements?

        (b) Charges reasonable and customary?

    (3) For care pre-authorized in Chapter 2-A-6, did any of these occur?

        (a) Did the HSWL SC assign a pre-authorization number?

        (b) Were services within the authorized, standard treatment plan?

        (c) Were treatments split to circumvent pre-authorization requirements?

    (4) For all dental services, do any of these apply?

        (a) Were services duplicated?

        (b) Were billings for the same service duplicated?

        (c) Were diagnosis charges consistent with services received?

        (d) Were crowns constructed of precious metals?

        (e) Are laboratory charges consistent with the service provided (bridges, crowns, partial or full dentures)?

f. Pharmacy.

    (1) For contract providers, were services within the scope of the contract?

    (2) For inpatient care, do any of these apply?

        (a) Were billings duplicated?

        (b) Was credit received for returned or unused medications?

(c) Did medication and in-patient dates coincide?

(d) Did medications' costs exceed 250 percent of Annual Pharmacists' Reference ("Red Book") average wholesale price (Note: This equals a 150 percent markup.)? Claims falling within ADCP guidelines are exempt from fee review.

CHAPTER 12

OCCUPATIONAL MEDICAL SURVEILLANCE AND
EVALUATION PROGRAM (OMSEP)

A. Information on the Occupational Medical Surveillance and Evaluation Program
is located in the Coast Guard Occupational Medicine Manual, COMDTINST
M6260.32 (series).

CHAPTER 13

QUALITY IMPROVEMENT

Chapter 13 Contents

CHAPTER THIRTEEN – QUALITY IMPROVEMENT

A. Quality Improvement Program.

1. Mission. The Commandant and Director of Health, Safety, and Work-Life are committed to providing the highest quality health care to Coast Guard beneficiaries. The Health Services Quality Improvement Program (QIP) outlined here establishes policy, prescribes procedures, and assigns responsibility for Quality Improvement (QI) activities at CG health services facilities. It is intended to function as an integral component in a quality healthcare system aimed at improving patient outcomes while also achieving patient satisfaction.

2. Internal Quality Assurance Reviews. The CG first established an internal healthcare quality assurance (QA) program in the early 1990s to monitor the quality of healthcare delivered at its clinics. The Maintenance and Logistics Command (MLC) administered the program by conducting QA surveys at each clinic. Clinics passing the MLC survey were awarded a three-year certificate that verified the clinic met CG health care operational requirements and QA standards. In 2004 the internal QA review process changed to the current format through which an external accreditation organization performs accreditation surveys of CG clinics and issues a one or three-year accreditation. To ensure CG specific operational requirements are maintained, a Health, Safety, and Work Life (HSWL) Service Center (SC) review process was developed to concentrate on CG-specific and Operational Health Readiness issues.

3. Healthcare Process Assessment Program (HPAP). CG specific QI and operational health readiness issues will be managed and monitored by the HSWL SC under the HPAP addressed in Chapter 13.D. The HSWL SC will no longer survey QA/QI issues that are addressed by the external accreditation surveyors nor provide a certification.

4. External Accreditation. The standard in the U.S. is for health care clinics to achieve and maintain external accreditation. Additionally, external accreditation allows the CG to meet DoD and TRICARE healthcare system requirements. In 2004, the CG contracted with an external accreditation organization to independently conduct CG clinic accreditation surveys. To receive a three-year accreditation, clinics must demonstrate compliance with current accreditation standards. A significant portion of the accreditation survey is focused on the quality of health care provided by the clinic, and the system to ensure continuous quality improvement is occurring.

5. Goals. The Institute of Medicine published six Aims for Improvement in their 2001 report, "Crossing the Quality Chasm". The Coast Guard embraces these aims within our health care program and our goals and objectives are developed to reflect that focus. Therefore, the Coast Guard strives to ensure healthcare is:

   a. Safe - avoiding injuries to patients from the care that is intended to help them.

   b. Effective - providing services based on scientific knowledge to all who could benefit and refraining from providing services to those not likely to benefit.

c. Patient-centered - providing care that is respectful of and responsive to individual patient preferences, needs, and values and ensuring the patient values guide all clinical decisions.

d. Timely - avoiding waits and sometimes harmful delays for both those who receive and those who give care.

e. Efficient - avoiding waste, including waste of equipment, supplies, ideas, and energy.

f. Equitable - providing care that does not vary in quality because of personal characteristics such as gender, geographic location, and socio-economic status.

6. Objectives. The framework to achieve our goals for quality healthcare is established through the following objectives:

a. Care is based on continuous healing relationships. Patients should receive care whenever they need it and in many forms, not just face to face visits. We will strive to be responsive at all times, and access to care will be provided through secure internet, by telephone, and other means as necessary to meet the need of our patients.

b. Care is customized according to patient needs and values. We will design our system to meet the most common needs of our patients, but we will strive to respond to individual patient choices and preferences.

c. The patient is the source of control. Patients will be given the necessary information and opportunity to exercise the degree of control they choose over health care decisions that affect them. We will strive to accommodate differences in patient preferences and encourage shared decision making.

d. Knowledge is shared and information flows freely. Clinicians and patients should communicate effectively and share information to enable quality care planning. Patients have access to their own medical information, and are encouraged to discuss treatment options with their provider.

e. Decision making is evidence based. We will strive to ensure patients receive care based on the best available scientific knowledge. This will include efforts to ensure the quality of care remains consistent across providers and locations.

f. Safety is a system property. We will strive to ensure patients are safe from injury caused by the care system. Reducing risk and ensuring safety will require greater attention to systems that help prevent and mitigate errors.

g. Needs are anticipated. Using population health information, we will strive to anticipate patient needs rather than react to events.

h. Waste is continuously decreased. We will review utilization practices as they relate to patient outcomes, and strive to ensure we do not waste resources or patient time.

i. Cooperation among clinicians is a priority. Clinicians and institutions should actively collaborate and communicate to ensure an appropriate exchange of information and coordination of care. We will strive to ensure continuity of patient care is optimized so that patient outcomes are improved.

7. Definitions.

   a. Quality. The desired level of performance as measured against generally accepted standards.

   b. Quality Health Care. As defined by the Institute of Medicine, quality health care is the degree to which health services for individuals and population increase the likelihood of desired health outcomes and are consistent with professional knowledge.

   c. Quality Assurance. The planned and systematic activities implemented in a system so that requirements for a product or service will be fulfilled. Quality Assurance activities include monitoring and evaluating based on established guidelines, e.g. laboratory quality control testing. Quality Assurance activities are designed to assure quality is maintained.

   d. Quality Improvement. Activities designed to raise the standards of the delivery of healthcare in order to maintain, restore or improve health outcomes of individuals and populations. Quality Improvement activities are interdisciplinary in nature and designed to continually assess and improve processes in the health care system.

   e. Quality Improvement Study (QIS). An assessment of patient care or clinic operations for the purpose of improvement through analysis, intervention, resolution, and follow up,

   f. Governing Body. A designated team that has authority and responsibility for improving the quality of patient care and providing organizational management and planning. This is the Commandant (CG-11) Executive Leadership Council. The Executive Leadership Council is comprised of Commandant (CG-112) (chair), Commandant (CG-11d), Commandant (CG-111), Commandant (CG-113), and HSWL SC.

8. Responsibilities.

   a. Director of Health, Safety, and Work-Life (CG-11).

      (1) Establish at all CG health care facilities a comprehensive QIP which meets industry standards published by independent accrediting organizations. The HSWL SC implements the QIP as established by the Director of Health and Safety.

      (2) Govern CG health care facilities with delegated responsibilities to the Senior Health Services Officer (SHSO) at each facility.

      (3) Establish and promulgate health care policy including professional performance standards against which quality can be measured.

(4) Establish and promulgate productivity and staffing standards for the health services program.

(5) Conduct periodic Quality Improvement Meetings for Headquarters and HSWL SC QI staffs to coordinate and implement program policy at all organizational levels.

(6) Review credentials and grant privileges for all CG medical and dental officers.

(7) Develop and promulgate the Quality Improvement Implementation Guides.

(8) Identify education and professional development training requirements and assure high quality standards are established and maintained. Coordinate and fund continuing professional education for all health services personnel.

b. Health, Safety, and Work-Life Service Center (HSWL SC).

(1) Ensure the Commandant's Health Care QI Program is executed at the field level.

(2) Periodically conduct site assist visits to ensure compliance with external accreditation organization standards and Healthcare Process Assessment Program (HPAP) goals of all health services facilities in their area in accordance with Chapter 13.D.

(3) Develop and maintain standard operating procedure manuals and/or health services support program guides necessary to provide operational guidance for clinic activities.

(4) Develop and maintain Quality Improvement Self Assessment Checklists for assist visits.

(5) Perform utilization review of clinic expenditures, staffing, equipment, supplies, and facilities; review and process all requests for non-Federal medical care from units in its jurisdiction.

(6) Provide technical and professional advice regarding health services to units, as required.

(7) Conduct site visits on an appropriate schedule to verify standards compliance and to provide assistance in meeting the expectations of the HPAP.

c. Commanding Officers.

(1) Ensure the unit actively pursues health services quality standards.

(2) Appoint in writing an individual to serve as Health Services Quality Improvement Coordinator.

d. Senior Health Services Officer (SHSO). Represents the Governing Body locally for Quality Improvement and related activities.

e. <u>Health Services QI Coordinator</u>. The Health Services QI Coordinator should be a senior health services staff member with these characteristics:

   (1) Demonstrates the ability and motivation to provide and ensure quality health care.

   (2) Knows the requirements of this Manual.

   (3) Clear in both written and oral communication.

   (4) Well versed in delivering CG health care and supports the goals of health care quality improvement.

   (5) Is an E-6 or above if military, or appropriate civilian employee.

f. <u>The Health Services QI Coordinator responsibilities</u>. The Health Services QI Coordinator responsibilities are as follows:

   (1) Directs Health Services QI Focus Group activities.

   (2) Implements the health care QI program locally by identifying and coordinating resolution of health care QI problems through design and implementation of QIS.

   (3) Develops and promulgates an annual QI calendar which sets the agenda for all QI activities at the unit, including among other activities QI Focus Group meetings and all quality improvement studies.

   (4) Other health care QI functions as necessary.

   (5) Appoint health services staff members to serve on a Health Services Quality Improvement Focus Group.

   (6) Forward copies of QI Focus Group meeting minutes to the HSWL SC.

g. <u>Alternate Health Services QI Coordinators</u>. The SHSO or Health Services Administrator may also be appointed as the Health Services QI Coordinator. However, this is not recommended in larger clinics since these two individuals are expected to provide necessary management expertise and clinical guidance in conducting the health care QI program and effecting any required program adjustments. The Health Services QI Coordinator's relationship to the SHSO is advisory.

h. <u>Accrediting Body</u>. An external accreditation organization that surveys CG clinics against nationally accepted standards. All facilities are expected to maintain compliance with current standards during the entire accreditation cycle. The regular accreditation cycle is three years.

i. <u>Less than 3 year certification</u>. Facilities that do not receive a three-year accreditation will be resurveyed within 12 months of the initial survey.

j. <u>Health Services Quality Improvement Focus Group (QIFG)</u>.

   (1) The Health Services QIFG shall consist of all clinic staff to a maximum of 15 members, depending on unit size, including both enlisted members and

officers who broadly represent the health care services provided at that unit.

(2) Members will include at least a medical or dental officer, a clinic supervisor, and department representatives, e.g., pharmacy, physical therapy, x-ray, and laboratory. If desired, the QIFG at small units may operate as a "Committee of the Whole" of all staff members.

(3) The QIFG advises the SHSO about the quality of the facility's health care and performs these functions:

(a) Identifies and resolves problems which affect the quality of health care delivery at the facility. The SHSO may delegate investigating and resolving a particular QI problem to the staff member responsible for the clinical area where the problem has been identified (e.g., laboratory, patient reception).

(b) Ensures all required health services committee meetings are held according to the provisions of the CG Medical Manual, HSWL SC standard operating procedures and operational guides, and local instructions, including, among others, the Patient Advisory Committee.

(c) Uses existing CG standards, HSWL SC self assessment checklists, and QIS to review and evaluate the quality of services delivered both in-house and by contract providers.

(d) Performs systematic, documented reviews of health records for compliance and adherence to Medical Manual standards and HSWL SC standard operating procedures, health and safety support program guides, self assessment checklists, and HIPAA privacy and security requirements.

(e) Solicits and monitors patient perceptions and satisfaction by surveys and questionnaires. Reports negative trends and potential solutions to the HSWL SC as a part of the QIFG meeting minutes.

(f) The QIFG shall meet at least quarterly and more often as local needs dictate. The clinic will maintain these meetings' original minutes for five years and will electronically forward copies of the minutes along with quality improvement studies through the chain of command to the HSWL SC for review on CG Central. The HSWL SC will provide electronic access to Commandant (CG-1122).

(g) Assists in obtaining and maintaining standards compliance necessary to achieve external accreditation.

9. <u>Confidentiality Statement</u>. All documents created under authority of the QI program are health services QI records and part of the CG's QIP. They are confidential and privileged under 14 USC 645 provisions. Releasing a health services QI document is expressly prohibited except in limited circumstances listed in 14 USC 645.

10. <u>QIP Review and Evaluation</u>. The Director of Health and Safety will annually review and evaluate the QIP. The review will reappraise the QI Plan and incorporate comments from the HSWL SC on implementation activities at field units during the preceding year.

    a. <u>QI Review and Evaluation Report</u>. By 30 November annually, HSWL SC shall provide to Commandant (CG-11) a written QI Review and Evaluation Report addressing these topics during the previous fiscal year:

        (1) Summary of clinic accreditations.

        (2) Summary of clinic HPAP compliance.

        (3) Summary of significant clinical problems identified.

        (4) Summary of peer review activities.

        (5) Recommended QIP modifications.

        (6) HSWL SC QI Plan for upcoming calendar year.

B. Credentials Maintenance and Review.

    1. Purpose. Verification of the authenticity of healthcare provider credentials/licensure is required to ensure appropriate preparation and qualification to engage in a specified scope of practice. Primary source verification is a mandatory step in the credentialing process. Credentials shall be verified for each healthcare provider appointed to a position providing patient care. Privileges are assigned based on this review.

    2. Responsibilities.

        a. Commandant (CG-11) is responsible for ensuring health care providers in CG facilities are qualified through proper credentialing.

        b. Commandant (CG-1122) must verify that credentials, including qualifying professional degree(s), license(s), graduate training, and references are valid before a provider may practice independently in CG health care facilities.

        c. Coast Guard providers (whether active duty, reserve, contract, or auxiliary) who provide direct patient care in CG health care facilities will comply with this chapter's provisions as applicable.

    3. Definitions.

        a. Allied Health Care Provider. A person who is trained to perform a health care task or service who is not listed as a provider and/or specifically named in this section by profession. An allied health care provider may hold a license, certification, or registration but generally does not initiate, modify, or terminate treatment independently. Allied health care providers include Independent Duty Health Services Technicians (IDHS), Health Services Technicians (HS), Nurses, Emergency Medical Technicians (EMT), Paramedics, Medical Assistants, Dental Technicians, Medical Technologists, or Lab Technicians.

        b. Auxiliarist. A medical or dental volunteer providing health care services to CG personnel in accordance with Coast Guard Auxiliarist Support to Coast Guard Health Care Facilities, COMDTINST 6010.2 (series).

        c. Centralized Credentials and Quality Assurance System (CCQAS). A worldwide web-based credential, risk management, and privileging application that enables the military healthcare system to manage clinician's credentials and privileging actions.

        d. Clinical Psychologist. A commissioned officer, civil service employee, or contract provider, who holds a Ph.D or Psy.D as a graduate of an accredited U.S. educational institution, has completed the required pre/post doctoral internships, and is licensed as a clinical psychologist.

        e. Contract Provider. An individual holding valid certification/licensure as a healthcare professional, who provides care in a CG Health Services facility under a contractual agreement with the CG. Contract providers are not considered medical or dental officers as it relates to duties and responsibilities.

f. Credentials. Documents constituting evidence of education, professional clinical training, licensure, experience, and expertise of a healthcare practitioner.

g. Credentials Maintenance. Filing, updating, modifying or completing files, documents and databases about practitioner credentials.

h. Credentials Review. The process of checking a practitioner's verified credentials and other supporting documents to evaluate potential assignments assign or rescind clinical privileges, or take administrative or personnel actions.

i. Credentials Verification. The process of verifying a practitioner's license, education, training, and competence before initial assignment or employment.

j. Credentials Verification Organization (CVO). An organization whose responsibilities include the collection, maintenance, and verification of healthcare provider credentials.

k. Dental Officer. A commissioned officer assigned to the CG, who is a graduate of a U.S. accredited school of dentistry and holds a valid, current, and unrestricted license to practice dentistry.

l. License (Current, Unrestricted, Active). A credential issued by one of the 50 states, District of Columbia or US Territories (Guam, Puerto Rico, Virgin Islands) that permits a person to practice medicine, dentistry, or other allied health profession.

m. Medical Officer.

    (1) A commissioned officer assigned to the CG who has graduated from a U.S. accredited educational institution and is currently licensed as a physician.

    (2) A Physician Assistant holding valid certification from the National Association on Certification of Physician Assistants (exempt from licensing requirement).

    (3) A Nurse Practitioner holding a valid certification by the American Academy of Nurse Practitioners or the American Nurses Credentialing Center.

n. Optometrist. A commissioned officer, civil service employee, or contractor who holds a doctor of Optometry degree as a graduate of a U. S. accredited educational institution, has completed the required internships, and licensed as an Optometrist.

o. <u>Pharmacist</u>.

    (1) <u>Pharmacy Officer</u>. A commissioned officer assigned to the CG who graduated from a U. S. accredited educational institution and is currently licensed as a pharmacist.

    (2) Contract Pharmacist. A contractor assigned to the CG who graduated from a U. S. accredited educational institution and is currently licensed as a pharmacist.

p. <u>Physical Therapist</u>. A commissioned officer, civil service employee, or contractor assigned to the CG who graduated from a U. S. accredited educational institution and is currently licensed as a physical therapist.

q. <u>Pre-selection Credentials Review</u>. The process of reviewing a practitioner's license, education, training, and competence before employment

r. <u>Primary Source Verification</u>. Verification of a credential by the CG CVO with an individual or institution possessing direct knowledge of the validity or authenticity of the particular credential.

s. <u>Privileges</u>. The practice activities authorized to be performed in the facility, within defined limits. Privileges are granted based on the providers' credentials and current competencies, as well as any facility limitations such as support staff and equipment.

t. <u>Provider</u>. A licensed and/or certified healthcare professional fully credentialed and in some cases granted individual clinical privileges to diagnose and treat diseases and conditions, including physicians, dentists, physician assistants, nurse practitioners, podiatrists, optometrists, and clinical psychologists, licensed clinical social workers, and licensed professional counselors.

4. <u>Pre-selection Credentials Review</u>.

a. <u>Commissioned Officers</u>. The PHS liaison officer at Commandant (CG-112), in cooperation with the PHS Division of Commissioned Corps Assignments (DCCA) in the Office of Commissioned Corps Operations (OCCO) shall perform a pre-employment review and verify minimum standards before recommending a CG detail for Commissioned personnel. DCCA also screens individuals and certain credentials as part of the commissioning process. CG procedures are designed to complement DCCAs; the CG may alter its policies to reflect OCCO policy changes.

b. <u>Civil Service Employees</u>. The HSWL SC or local command shall perform a pre-employment review of credentials for Civil Service employees providing care in CG health care facilities. Final credentialing is completed by the CG CVO.

c. <u>Contract Provider</u>. HSWL SC shall perform a pre-employment review of credentials for contractors providing care in CG health care facilities.

d. <u>Student credentials</u>. Commandant (CG-1122) will review and verify student credentials, as well as obtain a letter from the school stating the student's academic standing in accordance with Student Externship Programs, COMDTINST 6400.1 (series).

5. <u>Provider Credentials File (PCF)</u>. Files are developed and maintained by the CVO in Commandant (CG-1122). The CVO shall initiate and maintain PCFs for all Civil Service, Uniformed Service, Auxiliarist, and contracted providers for the entire length of their employment or service with CG. All credentials gathered for PCFs must be prime source verified and entered into the electronic credentialing system. Hard copy will also be maintained in paper files until otherwise determined by CG-11. For contract providers, the hiring entity (HSWL SC or HQ) will initiate the creation of the PCF (paper and electronic) through the CVO upon offer or intent to hire the provider. Persons unable or unwilling to provide required information may be disqualified for employment or accession. PCFs must contain the following credentials and supporting documentation:

a. <u>Curriculum vitae</u>. A curriculum vitae (CV) accounting for all time since the qualifying degree was received and prior to employment with the CG.

b. <u>Educational degrees</u>. Copies of qualifying educational degrees (diploma, certificate) needed to perform clinical duties with primary source verification.

c. <u>Postgraduate training certificates</u>. Copies of required postgraduate training certificates for the area of work; for example, internship, residency, fellowship, with primary source verification.

d. <u>State licenses</u>. Copies of state licenses for all states or territories in which the provider is licensed (active or inactive). The provider must maintain at least one unrestricted, current, and active license, and attach a statement of explanation for lapsed licenses or those subject to disciplinary action. All licenses must be primary source verified. Additionally, physicians must provide a copy of their Educational Commission for Foreign Medical Graduates (ECFMG) or United States Medical Licensing Examination (USMLE) certification if the provider graduated from a medical school not in the Continental US, Hawaii, Alaska, or from a medical school not accredited by the American Association Liaison Committee on Medical Education.

e. <u>Specialty board</u>. Copies of Coast Guard recognized specialty board and fellowship certificates with primary source verification of these documents. Coast Guard recognized specialty boards include American Board of Medical Specialties (ABMS), American Board of Physician Specialties (ABPS), National Commission on Certification of Physician Assistants (NCCPA), American Academy of Nurse Practitioners (AANP), or the American Nurses Credentialing Center (ANCC), and American Dental Association (ADA).

f. <u>Proof of competence and letters of reference</u>. Proof of current (within one year) competence, i.e., two letters of reference for initial appointment/accession and a description of recent clinical privileges held (practitioner's supervisor(s) from last five years must note concurrence with applicant's position, scope of practice and approval of privilege performance). Documents of reference submitted to DCCA for appointment in the USPHS may be used as letters of reference if these letters are within a 12 month period of CG detail.

g. Malpractice cases. A statement explaining any involvement in malpractice cases and claims, including a brief review of the facts about the practitioner's involvement.

h. Disciplinary action. A statement is needed explaining any disciplinary action from hospitals, licensing boards, or other agencies.

i. Basic Cardiac Life Support certification. A current Basic Cardiac Life Support (for Healthcare Providers), certification is required for all clinic personnel.

j. Advanced Cardiac Life Support. A current Advanced Cardiac Life Support certification is required for all active duty and reserve CG Medical Officers in accordance with Chapter 13 Section L of this Manual.

k. Drug Enforcement Agency (DEA). Copies of all current and prior Drug Enforcement Agency (DEA) registration, as appropriate.

l. National Practitioner Data Bank (NPDB). National Practitioner Data Bank (NPDB) query, current within two years.

m. Attestation Form.

n. Release of Information Letter.

o. National Provider Identifiers (NPI) Type 1.

6. Documentation.

a. Credential Documents. All credential documents must be sent to Commandant (CG-1122). Preference is for either scanned attachment to email or facsimile. Documents may also be sent via traceable means. The technical review by the HSWL SC does not constitute official Coast Guard credentialing or privileging.

b. Expiration of Credentials. It is ultimately the responsibility of the provider to ensure that all credentials required for clinical privileges are renewed prior to their expiration dates. If any credential required for clinical privileges is allowed to expire, the provider may have clinical privileges suspended or terminated. This will remove the provider from direct patient care and may render the provider ineligible to receive any special pay for clinical duties while the provider is in this status.

c. Confidentiality. The CVO will maintain files in a secure location. PCFs and their contents are Class III (maximum security) records and protected from disclosure. The Privacy Act (5 USC§552a) and the medical quality assurance confidentiality statute (14 USC§645) protect all documentation gathered in the credentialing process. Documents in the PCF will not be released to any other individual or entity unless the provider has given express written permission.

7. Electronic Credentialing System.

   a. In addition to the paper version PCF maintained with Commandant (CG-1122) CVO, provider credentials will also be entered into the CG Electronic Credentialing System. This web-based electronic system improves Commandant (CG-1122)'s ability to track credentials and see all credential information during the privileging process.

   b. Provider information entered into the CG Electronic Credentialing System is in accordance with provisions of the CG Health Services Quality Improvement Program. The Privacy Act (5 USC§552a) and the medical quality assurance confidentiality statute (14 USC§645) protect all documentation gathered in the credentialing process.

8. Verification.

   a. Credential verification. Education, training, licensure or registration, certification, ECFMG and board certification, must be verified by either an original letter from the educational institution or certifying body attesting to successful completion of specialty training. Verification may be printed from internet verification site, or verified by telephone call between the CVO representative and the educational institution or specialty board. In the case of telephone verification, record phone call and conversation on official letterhead signed and dated by the person making the call. Verification memo will include organization called, date, time, identify of call participants, and a detailed description of the call. Place all verification documents with their source documents in the PCF. Renewable credentials must be primary source verified upon receipt.

   b. Verify experience. Verification of experience and current competence requires at least two recommendation letters from appropriate sources as listed below. Commandant (CG-1122) CVO or the HSWL SC shall receive direct letters from the person providing the reference.

      (1) A letter either from the hospital chief of staff, clinic administrator, professional head, or department head if the individual has professional or clinical privileges or is associated with a hospital or clinic; or,

      (2) A letter from the director or a faculty member of the individual's training program if he or she has been in a training program in the previous two years.

9. Contract Provider Credentials Review.

   a. Contracting agency. The contracting agency has the responsibility for initial and ongoing primary source verification of credentials of all contract providers. Physician Assistants must be certified by the National Commission on Certification of Physician Assistants. Nurse Practitioners must be certified by the American Academy of Nurse Practitioners or the American Nurses

Credentialing Center. Malpractice insurance must be provided and verified by the contracting agency.

b. Technical review. At the contracting officer's request, HSWL SC will perform a technical review of the providers' credentials. This does not constitute a privileging authorization.

10. Reverification.

a. Renewable credentials. These credentials are renewable and will be primary source verified on renewal: License, PA certification, Board certification, and contract providers' malpractice coverage. Reverify contract providers' updated credentials is at contract renewal.

b. Reverify these credentials by original letter or telephone contact. The person making the call will record telephone contact on the document or by a separate, signed memorandum.

11. National Practitioner Data Bank (NPDB).

a. Commandant's role. Commandant (CG-11) possesses sole authority to report to the NPDB. Commandant (CG-1122) is designated as the appropriate entity for all NPDB queries. Coordinate all queries for patient care providers through this branch.

b. NPDB requirements. A reply from the NPDB is not required before the practitioner begins providing services. However, any provider whose credential verification is not fully completed will be considered to have a conditional appointment until all credentials are verified as required.

12. National Provider Identifiers Type 1 (NPI).

a. Requirement for NPI. All health care providers who furnish health care services or those who may initiate and/or receive referrals must obtain an NPI Type 1. NPI Type 1 is assigned at no fee by the Centers for Medicare and Medicaid Services (CMS) National Plan and Provider Enumeration System (NPPES). Providers shall apply for and will receive one and only one NPI Type 1. This NPI Type 1 will be a permanent identifier. CMS has an on-line NPI Type 1 application available at https://nppes.cms.hhs.gov.

b. Filing the NPI. Once a provider obtains their NPI Type 1, they shall provide a copy to the CG credentialing office, Commandant (CG-1122). The information will be entered into the Centralized Credentials Quality Assurance System (CCQAS) database. A photocopy of the original hardcopy will be filed in the Practitioner Credentials File.

c. Instructions. Instructions for obtaining and maintaining NPI Type 1 for health care providers are to be included in all privileging packages.

d. HIPAA compliance. HIPAA compliance requires that NPPES be updated within 30 days of a change in the NPI Type 2 data.

e. Privileging authority facility name. In order to ensure standardized addresses are being used in the mailing address and in the practice location fields on the

NPI Type 1 application, providers (other than Reserve component providers) are to use the privileging authority facility name (USCG HQ, COMMANDANT (CG-1122)) as the address of record.

C. Clinical Privileges.

1. Purpose. Clinical privileges define the provider's scope of care and services available to patients. The privileging process is directed solely and specifically at providing quality patient care; it is not a disciplinary or personnel management system. However, privileging actions may accompany administrative or judicial actions or engender them. Granting and rescinding clinical privileges is highly confidential, and must be conducted according to strict rules to prevent improper or prejudiced actions. This section establishes processes and procedures to grant and rescind clinical privileges. These provisions fall outside the scope of the Administrative Investigations Manual, COMDTINST M5830.1 (series).

2. Applicability and Scope. All uniformed, Civil Service, contract civilian, and auxiliarist CG health care providers shall have clinical privileges assigned. Health Services personnel (other than providers) who function under a standard job or position description or standard protocol, policies, and procedures, or who must consult with another provider before or during medical or dental treatment will not receive clinical privileges.

3. Definitions.

   a. Abeyance. The temporary assignment of a health care provider from clinical to non-clinical duties while an internal or external peer review or quality assurance investigation or action is conducted. Periods of abeyance provide privileging authorities the opportunity to review allegations while ensuring patient safety and protecting providers from unwarranted adverse privileging action. An abeyance terminates upon referral to a peer review hearing or at the end of 28 days, whichever occurs sooner. An abeyance is not an adverse action and is non-punitive.

   b. Adverse Privileging Action. Denying, suspending, restricting, reducing, or revoking clinical privileges based upon misconduct, professional impairment, or lack of professional competence. The termination of professional staff appointment based upon conduct incompatible with continued professional staff membership may also result in an adverse privileging action.

   c. Clinical Privileges. Type of practice activities authorized to be performed in the facility, within defined limits, based on the providers' education, professional license as appropriate, experience, current competence, ability, judgment, and health status.

   d. Core Privileges. Standard set of practice activities authorized and expected to be performed by any privileged provider within designated categories.

   e. Convening Authority. Official that grants provider privileges and directs the meeting of the Special Professional Review Committee (SPRC). For Coast Guard Health Services, the convening authority is Commandant (CG-11).

   f. Document Review. A review of medical record documentation and other pertinent data as defined by the Convening Authority.

g. <u>External Review</u>. Administrative, non-judicial, or criminal investigations initiated by entities other than the CG health services program. External reviews may be conducted by an outside agency only in accordance with 5 USC 552a The Privacy Act and 14 USC 645 Medical Quality Assurance Documents Confidentiality.

h. <u>Focused Review</u>. An internal administrative mechanism to evaluate information about clinical care or practice. CG health services officers conduct focused reviews as part of the quality improvement program.

i. <u>Full Staff Privileges</u>. Core or Core and Supplemental privileges granted for a full term by the Convening Authority.

j. <u>Impairment</u>. Any personal characteristic or condition that may adversely affect the ability of a health care provider to render quality care. Impairments may be professional, behavioral, or medical.

   (1) Professional impairments include deficits in medical knowledge, expertise, or judgment.

   (2) Behavioral impairments include unprofessional, unethical, or criminal conduct.

   (3) Medical impairments are conditions that impede or preclude a health care provider from safely executing his or her responsibilities as a health care provider.

k. <u>Initial Staff Privileges</u>. Core or Core and Supplemental privileges granted to a provider that has not previously been granted privileges with the Coast Guard. Privileges are granted for one year while a review of proficiencies and suitability is conducted.

l. <u>National Practitioner Data Bank (NPDB)</u>. The agency established per regulations issued by the Department of Health and Human Services to collect and maintain data on substandard clinical performance and unprofessional conduct of health care providers. Requires reports of adverse privileging actions taken against providers and payments made to settle or satisfy claims or judgments resulting from medical malpractice of providers.

m. <u>Peer Review</u>. Review by an individual (or individuals) who possess relevant professional knowledge or experience, usually in the same discipline as the individual under review.

n. <u>Privileging</u>. The granting of permission and responsibility for a healthcare provider to provide specified or delineated healthcare within the scope of their licensure, certification, or registration. Clinical privileges define the scope and limits of practice for individual providers and are based on the capability of the healthcare facility, licensure, relevant training and experience.

o. <u>Privileging Authority</u>. Individual who ultimately authorizes privileges based on recommendations by the Professional Review Committee (PRC). Director, Health, Safety, and Work-Life, Commandant (CG-11) is the corporate privileging authority for all CG health care providers.

COMDTINST M6000.1F

p. Professional Review Committee (PRC). A committee appointed by Commandant (CG-11) to review credentials and supporting documentation with respect to requests for clinical privileges and make recommendations for action to the Privileging Authority. The committee shall be composed of the Deputy Director of Health, Safety and Work-Life, Commandant (CG-11d), the Chief of Operational Medicine and Medical Readiness, Commandant (CG-1121), and the Chief of Quality Performance and Improvement Division, Commandant (CG-1122) or their designees. The committee shall have at least two Medical Officers (one of which shall be a physician and the other may be a PA or NP) and one Dental Officer. Other officers may participate as required (e.g. Auxiliarist Medical Officer).

q. Provider. An individual granted clinical privileges to independently examine, diagnose, and treat diseases and conditions within their scope of licensure, certification, or registration. Physicians, dentists, physician assistants, nurse practitioners and other professions so designated by the privileging authority are provider disciplines within the CG health services program.

r. Provisional Privileges. A non-adverse decision to grant privileges to a previously privileged provider for a specified period of time pending further review and approval of full privileges by the PRC.

s. Special Professional Review Committee. An ad hoc Professional Review Committee independent of the PRC, specifically designated by the Convening Authority to address allegation and/or complaints regarding a CG provider.

t. Summary of Suspension. The temporary removal of all or part of a provider's clinical privileges during the completion of due process procedures. A summary of suspension is used during the period between an abeyance and the completion of due process procedures. Summary of suspension of privileges is not reportable to the NPDB unless the final action is reportable.

u. Supplemental Privileges. Practice activities, in addition to the core privileges, that may be requested and granted based on needs and capabilities of the facility, and skills and ability of the requesting provider as authorized by the privileging authority.

v. Suspension. The temporary removal of all or part of a provider's clinical privileges after due process procedures are completed. In such cases, the NPDB must be notified of the suspension, and then informed when privileges are reinstated, or if not reinstated, when privileges are reduced or revoked.

4. Clinical Privileges.

a. General.

(1) Commandant (CG-11) will take privileging actions based on recommendations of the PRC. When reviewing supplemental privilege requests, Commandant (CG-11) shall consider limitations (facility, support staff, equipment capability, etc.), which may prevent a provider from conducting certain activities. Commandant (CG-11) shall assign

Chapter 13. C. Page 3

providers to perform professional duties only if their education, training, and experience qualify them to perform such duties. Commandant (CG-11) shall also consider the provider's health status and ability to treat coworkers and patients with dignity and respect when granting privileges.

(2) Requests for clinical privileges will be generated in the electronic privileging system. If supplemental privileges are requested, supporting documentation verifying the training and experience for requested privileges must accompany the request for supplemental privileges. Requests will be reviewed by the appropriate supervisors and force managers before presentation at the PRC meeting. The PRC shall review the privileges requested and make a recommendation to Commandant (CG-11). The recommendations of the PRC will not be considered final until Commandant (CG-11) approves them. A provider shall not be granted access authority in the Electronic Health Record (EHR) or other EHR type databases until their privileges have been approved by Commandant (CG-11).

(3) Absence of clinical privileges must not delay treatment in an emergency (a situation in which failure to provide treatment would result in undue suffering or endanger life or limb). In such cases the providers are expected to do everything in their power to save patients.

(4) On transfer, the provider shall retain core privileges, but must request any supplemental privileges supported by the gaining facility.

(5) When providers with full staff privileges in the CG are assigned TAD outside their respective field office for greater than 90 days, the TAD orders issuing authority shall request that Commandant (CG-1122) transmit a copy of the provider's clinical privileges to the host SME/SDE who will evaluate the privileges and advise the provider if any supplemental privileges will be authorized at that site. Any change to privileges based on facility limitations is not considered an adverse action.

(6) When providers from DoD are assigned TAD to CG clinics, their parent command shall transmit an Inter-agency Credentials Transfer Brief (ICTB) and a copy of their clinical privileges to the host command prior to their arrival. The SME/SDE will determine if all privileges are appropriate and shall contact Commandant (CG-1122) for clarification where needed. Any change to privileges based on facility limitations is not considered an adverse action.

b. Procedures.

(1) The CG PHS liaison in Commandant (CG-112) will inform prospective PHS providers assigned to the CG that they must request clinical privileges in writing before accession to active duty or formal employment.

(2) The PRC will recommend initial privileges for all providers new to the Coast Guard. Providers may request full staff privileges after this initial performance period.

(3) The PRC will evaluate full staff privileges every **three years**. Commandant (CG-1122) CVO shall give notice to providers when privileges are due to expire. Providers will submit privilege requests to Commandant (CG-1122) CVO at least 90 days before privileges are due for renewal.

(4) Although Commandant (CG-1122) will provide notice of renewal, it is ultimately the responsibility of the provider to ensure they maintain current credentials and privileges at all times. Current credentials and privileges are considered a condition of employment, therefore, expiration of credentials or privileges may result in an inability to provide patient care, which will also affect the ability to renew special pay contracts.

(5) In the event that a new request for privileges has not arrived at Commandant (CG-1122) within 30 days of the current privileges expiration date, a letter/e-mail will be forwarded to the SME/SDE and the provider, with a copy to the HSWL SC, notifying them that the provider's current privileges are due to expire in 30 days, and when expired the provider will no longer be allowed to provide patient care.

c. Routine Operations of the Professional Review Committee (PRC).

(1) Commandant (CG-1122) is responsible for monitoring and administering the privileging process for all providers in the Health Services program that require clinical privileges to perform their duties.

(2) The PRC will make recommendations to Commandant (CG-11) on the granting of clinical privileges.

(3) The PRC may also be convened by Commandant (CG-11) to review PCFs for situations other than the routine review of clinical privileges.

(4) Commandant (CG-1122) CVO will forward requests for clinical privileges as well as the PCFs, to the cognizant Force Manager who will evaluate the PCFs and decide if the request should be presented before the PRC or if further information or action is required before submission to the PRC.

(5) The PRC will evaluate each PCF and recommend any of the following actions for each case:

(a) Grant all requested privileges as either initial or full.

(b) Hold privileges in abeyance for providers with expired credentials until credentials are updated and current.

(c) Request any decision regarding privileges be deferred until additional supporting information is submitted to the PRC.

(d) Maintain or modify current privileges while more information is forthcoming or an investigation is being conducted.

(e) Request a focused review or other type of internal investigation.

(f) Request an external review or investigation.

(g) Other actions as dictated by circumstances.

(6) The PRC will discuss each case but the decision to recommend approval or rejection of a privileging action will be made by Commandant (CG-11d).

(7) The PRC will forward its recommendations for privileging actions in the minutes of the meeting to Commandant (CG-11).

    (a) Commandant (CG-1122) will prepare the minutes for each meeting of the PRC.

    (b) The minutes will specify the recommended privileging action.

    (c) In the event of a recommendation by the PRC for any privileging action less than granting full privileges, the minutes shall specify the reasons or justification for that recommendation.

(8) After receiving the minutes, Commandant (CG-11) will make a decision on the recommendations of the PRC. In cases where the PRC has recommended the granting of full privileges, the Request for Clinical Privileges will be submitted to Commandant (CG-11) for final approval.

d. <u>Non Routine Privileging Actions</u>.

(1) All actions and processes on granting, reducing, suspending, and revoking clinical privileges are conducted in accordance with provisions of the CG health services Quality Improvement Program. The Privacy Act (5 USC§552a) and the medical quality assurance confidentiality statute (14 USC§645) protect all documentation related to these processes.

(2) Actions to review, reduce, or withdraw clinical privileges will be taken promptly if reasonable cause exists to doubt a provider's competence to practice or for any other cause affecting patient safety. Reasonable cause includes: a grossly negligent single incident; a pattern either of inappropriate prescribing or substandard of care; an incompetent or negligent act causing death or serious bodily injury; abuse of legal or illegal drugs or diagnosis of provider substance dependence; practitioner disability (physical and/or mental psychiatric conditions(s) impairing clinical duties); or a provider's significant unprofessional conduct. In such cases, notification will be provided to Commandant (CG-11) immediately.

(3) Regional Practice Manager (in consultation with Regional Practice SME/SDE, as appropriate) will review all complaints related to providers that originate at the local clinic or practice level. If a reasonable cause exists to doubt a provider's competence, or in the event of allegations of substandard or improper medical or dental treatment by a provider occurring in a CG health care facility, notification containing the allegations shall be immediately forwarded to the HSWL SC. In cases

where notification originates from military members or organizations, transmittal shall be via their chain of command to the HSWL SC.

(4) The HSWL SC will review all provider related complaints with the designated Force Manager (FM). The FM will assess complaint and bring to the PRC with any other background information deemed applicable by the FM.

(5) The PRC will review the complaint and may choose to either request a more detailed review from HSWL SC, or to forward to the Convening Authority for further action.

(6) Upon review of allegations, the Convening Authority shall, within 5 working days, designate appropriate follow-up action or disposition that may include the appointment of a Special Professional Review Committee (SPRC). The Convening Authority shall designate the composition of the SPRC when one is appointed.

(7) Once appointed, the SPRC shall convene and complete all review within a time not to exceed 15 working days. After reviewing the allegations, the SPRC shall make recommendations to the Convening Authority that may include: a focused review team, a documentation review, or other disposition as appropriate.

(8) Based on the nature of the allegation(s) and the recommendations of the SPRC, the Convening Authority may order a focused review team (on-site), a document review, or other disposition. In cases requiring further review, the Convening Authority will designate focused review team members or the document review officer through the HSWL SC within 10 working days from receipt of the SPRC's recommendation, and shall further define the particular review process based upon the nature of the allegations giving rise to the review.

(9) The focused review team or document reviewing officer shall initiate and complete the review action within 30 working days after the Convening Authority designates the review action.

(10) If the provider under review is a physician, the focused review team shall consist of at least three CG physicians. If the provider under review is a Flight Surgeon, Aviation Medical Officer (AMO), or Aeromedical Physician Assistant at least one of the reviewing physicians must be a Flight Surgeon. For a Dental Officer, the reviewing team shall consist of at least three CG Dental Officers. For a physician assistant or nurse practitioner, the team shall consist of three Medical Officer reviewers; one of which must be a physician assistant or nurse practitioner as applicable. The Convening Authority may assign additional team members (not to exceed 5 total team members) to assist in the review process.

(11) In cases requiring a document review officer, the HSWL SC, shall take measures to ensure the document review officer is impartial and will not represent any conflict of interest. The document review officer shall be of the

same discipline as the provider under review, however, when the provider being reviewed is a Physician Assistant or Nurse Practitioner the document review officer may be a physician.

(12) The provider under review need not be present for records or other document review, but when possible should be available to answer questions for the focused review team or document review officer.

(13) The document review officer or focus review team shall brief the unit CO about significant findings at the end of the visit. Within 10 working days of concluding the review, the Convening Authority shall receive a written report for disposition containing findings, conclusions and specific recommendations, through the HSWL SC.

(14) Focused review team or document review reports shall contain at least one of these recommendations:

(a) No action.

(b) Administrative action, such as verbal counseling.

(c) Reassignment to another facility for observation, supervision, and/or additional training (may or may not involve reduction of privileges).

(d) Privilege reappraisal.

(e) Reduction of privileges (specify extent of reduction).

(f) Privilege suspension (indefinite).

(g) Permanent removal from clinical duties (privilege revocation).

(h) Further review.

(15) If the document review officer or focused review team recommends immediate adverse privileging action, they shall contact the Convening Authority by the most expedient means possible.

(16) Upon review of the written report, the Convening Authority shall within three working days, determine further disposition that may include reconvening the SPRC for further review and recommendations. In the event that the written report recommends adverse privileging action, the Convening Authority shall reconvene the SPRC for further review and recommendations.

(17) If reconvened, the SPRC shall review all available records, may contact potential witnesses to assist in their deliberation, and shall provide recommendations to the Convening Authority within 30 working days.

(18) If the SPRC recommends adverse privileging action, the Commandant (CG-112) Office Chief shall contact the provider under review the same duty day if possible, either by phone or in person. Written notification will be sent to the provider under review within five working days via traceable means which shall include notification that an adverse privileging action has been recommended against him or her

and the reasons for the proposed action. The written notice shall further delineate that the provider has a right to request an appeal on the proposed action and the time limit (up to 30 working days) within which to request such an appeal in writing and specify the provider's rights in the appeal process.

(19)   The provider's failure to request or appear at the appeal, absent good cause, constitutes a waiver of further appeal and appeal rights, and the proposed adverse privileging action shall be finalized by the Convening Authority.

(20)   In the case where an adverse privileging action becomes final, all adverse privileging actions that restrict or suspend clinical privileges for longer than 30 days will be reported to the National Practitioner Data Bank (NPDB). Providers may dispute Data Bank information as provided in 45 CFR 60, "National Practitioner Data Bank for Adverse Information on Physicians and Other Health Care Practitioners."

e. Appeal Process.

(1)   If a provider requests a hearing in writing within the time limit, Commandant (CG-112) shall within 10 working days schedule the appeal hearing. Notification of the appeal hearing to the provider must state the hearing place, time, and date; which shall be convened not less than 30 days but not longer than 60 days after the date the written request for an appeal hearing was received by Commandant (CG-112). The provider will also be given a written list of witnesses (if any) expected to testify at the hearing on behalf of the hearing committee.

(2)   Commandant (CG-112) will assign the hearing committee, consisting of three CG/PHS officers equivalent or higher in rank to the provider under review, not previously involved in the internal review process. The disciplines represented shall be the same as required for the focused review team. Each hearing committee member will have one vote.

(3)   The provider under review has these rights:

(a)   To consult with CG legal counsel or civilian legal counsel at his/her own expense. While such counsel may attend the hearing and advise the provider during the proceedings, the counsel will not be allowed to participate directly in the hearing, (e.g., may not ask questions, respond to questions on behalf of the provider, or seek to enter material into the record).

(b)   To obtain a transcript of the proceedings by paying any reasonable preparation charges.

(c)   To call, examine, and cross-examine witnesses. The provider is responsible for arranging the presence of his or her witnesses and failure of the witnesses to appear will not constitute a procedural error or basis for delaying the proceedings.

(d) To present relevant verbal or written evidence regardless of its admissibility in a court of law.

(e) To submit a written statement at the close of the hearing.

(4) The hearing committee shall review all relevant records, hear all witnesses, and have the right to interview all witnesses. The hearing committee shall request assistance from Commandant (CG-0944) throughout the hearing process.

(5) The hearing committee will base its recommendation on whether or not to sustain, reduce, suspend, or revoke a provider's clinical privileges on a preponderance of the evidence as judged by a majority vote. A report of the hearing committee's final recommendations will be reported to the Convening Authority within two working days after the hearing ends.

(6) The Convening Authority will review the hearing committee's recommendations within three working days of receiving their report; make a decision and notify the provider under review the day of the decision either by telephone or in person; and send written notice to the provider by DHS authorized commercial traceable means, within five working days after the hearing ends. The Convening Authority's decision shall be final.

D. Healthcare Process Assessment Program (HPAP).

1. Purpose. The primary mission of the CG clinics is to maintain the operational health readiness of active duty and reserve personnel by assuring their availability to physically and mentally meet worldwide deployment standards in accordance with this Manual. Maintaining a high level of health readiness involves collaboration between providers, commands, clinics and the HSWL SC. HPAP is designed to provide a framework to ensure all clinics monitor and comply with CG specific healthcare-related requirements not reviewed through external accreditation.

2. Overview.

   a. Program Elements. The HPAP is designed for clinics to monitor those healthcare-related QA and operational issues not reviewed by external surveyors and to ensure units within their area-of-responsibility (AOR) are operationally ready in accordance with CG standards. There are three issues that require oversight.

      (1) Coast Guard specific QA items reviewed by HSWL SC not covered through external accreditation.

      (2) Coast Guard specific policies and procedures affecting operational health readiness in the AOR.

      (3) Coast Guard specific clinic administrative operations and requirements such as financial management activities.

   b. Monitoring the HPAP. Clinics must review the operational health readiness of active duty/reserve members within their AORs on a regular basis. It is the Command's responsibility to ensure medical and dental readiness of the active duty/reserve members in their AOR. It is the responsibility of the SHSO to develop and maintain a plan that ensures optimal health readiness for all active duty/reserve members within the designated AOR in accordance with guidance provided in this instruction. The HSWL SC will review CG-specific QA and operational health readiness issues on a continual basis and provide needed assistance to clinics to ensure a high level of health readiness. Healthcare process compliance will be accomplished through reviews of each individual clinic's information posted in HPAP databases, QA public folders on CG Central and the HSWL SC assist visits. A post-visit HPAP evaluation report will be provided to the clinics through the CO.

   c. Accreditation. The HPAP does not confer accreditation or certification status. Operational readiness is a command-directed process. The HSWL SC provides assistance in meeting HPAP goals, QA/QI standards and preparation for the external accreditation survey.

3. HPAP Compliance Process.

   a. Responsibility.

      (1) Unit. The unit CO is responsible for ensuring the command's health care facility complies with standards set forth in this Manual and the HSWL SC HPAP.

COMDTINST M6000.1F

(2) <u>Clinics</u>. The SHSO is responsible for routinely monitoring the progress of medical, dental, pharmacy readiness within their AOR and the implementation of the HPAP.

(3) <u>HSWL SC</u>. Responsible for developing and coordinating process checklists, self-assessment tools, assist visits to the clinics, and process reviews

(4) <u>Headquarters</u>. Chief, Directorate of Health, Safety, and Work-Life coordinates and directs the program, adjudicates appeals, and promulgates appropriate standards governing CG delivery of health care and policies on managing and operating CG health care facilities.

b. <u>Process Checklist</u>. The process checklists show QA and/or operational readiness tasks that clinics must address on a regular basis. The checklists are not all-inclusive because they do not list tasks that do not directly apply to QA or operational readiness (e.g. "take out trash"). Clinics must determine what tasks they do on a regular basis and have mechanisms in place to ensure these tasks get completed. The HSWL SC will assist in this effort. To view the most current HPAP compliance checklist go to the HSWL SC microsite on CG Central.

c. <u>Self-Assessment</u>. Health readiness and policy adherence is a continuous process and must be routinely reviewed by the clinic and HSWL SC. Self-assessment tools serve as a guide to assess how well the intent of the HPAP is being met through the daily operations of the clinic. Clinics that are diligent in addressing the issues listed on the self-assessment sheets should meet AAAHC QI and CG HPAP standards.

d. <u>Quality Improvement Studies (QISs)</u>. Clinics must demonstrate that they have a system in place to monitor healthcare delivery. Previously this was done through retroactive data reviews of given topics (i.e. monitoring and evaluation reports). With external accreditation, clinics must review areas of concern or interest and implement quality improvement studies. QISs may be adapted for operational readiness or other issues not reviewed by the external accreditation organization.

e. <u>CG Central</u>. CG Central serves as the primary repository for HPAP QA/QI documents such as QIFG meeting minutes, SOPs, and Letters of Designation, and other items listed on Quality Improvement Calendar, Form CG-6000-5.

f. <u>Public QA/QI Folders</u>. Public folders may be used for depositing QA/QI documents (e.g. CBRN antidote inventories) but do not take the place of using CG Central.

E. Quality Improvement Implementation Guide (QIIG).

1. Purpose. The QIIG is a series of exercises designed to assist commands in meeting Health Services QI Program requirements and to augment policy that is outlined in the Medical Manual. Serving as a guideline, the QIIG minimizes the QI program administrative requirements by providing direction and, in many cases, templates for addressing critical quality issues. The exercises facilitate clinic efforts to develop local policies and procedures by providing generic frameworks clinics can adapt to local conditions. In some cases, clinics may be required to submit evidence of completing an exercise to the HSWL SC for data evaluation purposes.

2. Responsibilities.

    a. Commandant (CG-112). Commandant (CG-112) develops exercises as needed on critical quality issues for inclusion in the QIIG and posts them on http://www.uscg.mil/hq/cg1/cg112/cg1122/QIIG.asp.

    b. HSWL SC. HSWL SC ensures exercises are available to Commands for clinic personnel to complete and also reviews clinic's use of the QIIGs as part of the Healthcare Process Assessment Program.

    c. Unit QI Coordinator. Unit QI Coordinators ensure staff promptly complete all QIIG exercises and maintain a complete, updated QIIG folder.

F. National Provider Identifiers.

1. <u>National Provider Identifiers (NPI) Type 1 (NPI)</u>.

   a. <u>Who must have a Type 1 NPI</u>. All health care providers who provide health care services or those who may initiate and/or receive referrals must obtain an NPI Type 1. A NPI Type 1 is assigned at no fee by the Centers for Medicare and Medicaid Services (CMS) National Plan and Provider Enumeration System (NPPES). Providers shall apply for and will receive one and only one NPI Type 1. This NPI Type 1 will be a permanent identifier unique to that provider. CMS has an online NPI Type 1 application available at https://nppes.cms.hhs.gov.

   b. <u>Copies of the NPI</u>. Once a provider obtains their NPI Type 1 they shall provide a copy to Commandant (CG-1122). The information will be entered into the Centralized Credentials Quality Assurance System (CCQAS) database. A photocopy of the original hardcopy will be filed in the Practitioner Credentials File.

   c. <u>Obtaining and maintaining a NPI</u>. Instructions for obtaining and maintaining NPI Type 1 for health care providers are to be included in all privileging packages.

   d. <u>Updates</u>. HIPAA compliance requires that NPPES be updated within 30 days of a change in the NPI Type 1 data. (Example: provider changes their name or provider changes their duty station).

   e. <u>Privileging authority address</u>. In order to ensure standardized addresses are being used in the mailing address and in the practice location fields on the NPI Type 1 application, providers (other than Reserve component providers) are to use the privileging authority facility name (USCG HQ, Commandant (CG-1122)) as the address of record.

2. <u>Clinic National Provider Identifiers (NPI) Type 2</u>.

   a. <u>Who must have a NPI Type 2</u>. Per the HIPAA NPI Final Rule, 45 CFR, Part 162, all health care facilities that provide health care services must have an NPI Type 2. The NPI Type 2s are assigned at no fee by the CMS and NPPES. CMS has an online NPI Type 2 application available at https://nppes.cms.hhs.gov.

   b. <u>SHSO</u>. Each SHSO is responsible for submitting the initial NPI application and updates. Once a clinic obtains their NPI Type 2 they shall provide a copy to Commandant (CG-1122). The clinic shall maintain the NPI Type 2 in a permanent record.

   c. <u>Updates</u>. HIPAA compliance requires that NPPES be updated within 30 days of a change in the NPI Type 2 data. (Example: Address change).

G. Health Insurance Portability and Accountability Act (HIPAA).

   1. Background.

      a. Health Insurance Portability and Accountability Act, (HIPAA). The Health Insurance Portability and Accountability Act, (HIPAA), was signed into law as Public Law 104-191 on 21 August 1996. The purpose of the law includes efforts to improve health insurance portability and renewability, combat fraud and abuse, promote medical liability reform, and simplify the administration of health insurance. Title II, Subtitle F on Administrative Simplification required the Secretary of Health & Human Service to publish standards for electronic exchange, privacy and security of health information.

      b. Federal Regulations. The promulgated regulations, known as the Privacy Rule are found at 45 Code of Federal Regulations (CFR) Part 160 and Part 164, Subparts A and E. The Security Rule is found at 45 CFR Part 164, Subpart C. These regulations became effective as of April 21, 2003, and compliance was required as of April 21, 2006. These regulations are available at the following web sites:

        (1) http://www.hhs.gov/ocr/privacy/hipaa/understanding/summary/ or

        (2) Parallel **Defense Health Agency (DHA)**/Department of Defense implementing regulations are found at: **http://health.mil/Military-Health-Topics/Privacy-and-Civil-Liberties/Privacy-Act-and-HIPAA-Privacy-Training**.

   2. HIPAA Privacy/Security Officials (P/SO). 45 C.F.R. § 164.530(a) requires (1) the designation of a privacy official responsible for the development and implementation of policies and procedures and (2) the designation of a contact person who is responsible for receiving complaints and providing further information about matters covered under the Notice of Privacy Practices. 45 C.F.R. § 164.308(a) (2) requires that the CG "identify the security official who is responsible for the development and implementation of the policies and procedures required by this subpart for the entity."

      a. The CG HIPAA Privacy and Security **Officers**.

        (1) The Chief, Office of Health Services, Commandant (CG-112) shall designate an officer as the CG Privacy Officer, residing within Commandant (CG-112). This officer shall serve as the Privacy Officer (PO) for the CG Health Care System and as the CG Service Representative to the DHA Privacy Office. The CG HIPAA Security Officer, residing in Commandant (CG-114), Office of Health, Safety and Work-Life Business Operations, will serve as the Security Officer for the CG Health Care system. Primary responsibilities will be to establish, modify, and disseminate CG HIPAA security policy.

        (2) Responsibilities of the **CG PO** are:

(a) Provide coordination between the CG and **DHA** Privacy Office on all HIPAA related issues.

(b) Maintain current knowledge of applicable Federal and State privacy laws, accreditation standards and CG regulations. Monitor advancements in emerging privacy and health information security technologies to ensure that the Coast Guard is positioned to adapt and comply with these advancements.

(c) Establish, modify and disseminate CG HIPAA policy.

(d) Serve as the CG HIPAA liaison to receive complaints and provide further information about matters covered by the notice required by the HIPAA Privacy Rule, 45 CFR Parts 160 and 164, from Health and Human Services (HHS), **DHA**, and Congress.

(e) Serve as the local P/SO for the Commandant (CG-11).

b. <u>HSWL-Service Center (SC) HIPAA Privacy and Security Officer</u>.

(1) The Commanding Officer, Health Safety Work Life (HSWL) Service Center (SC), shall designate a junior officer as the HSWL-SC P/SO for the CG Health Care System.

(2) Responsibilities of the HSWL-SC P/SO are:

(a) Serve as the CG HIPAA liaison to receive complaints and provide further information about matters covered by the HIPAA Privacy Rule, 45 CFR Parts 160 and 164, from all Coast Guard commands and all HSWL clinic P/SOs.

(b) Maintain a log of all local HSWL clinic P/SOs and a file of all letters of designation.

(c) Develop Standard Operating Procedures (SOPs) for clinic practice implementation of the HIPAA Privacy and Security Regulation requirements.

(d) Establish and recognize best practices relative to the management of the privacy and security of health information.

(e) Serve as a liaison to other P/SOs.

(f) Review all system-related information security plans throughout the local health care network to ensure alignment between security and privacy practices, and act as liaison to the information systems department.

(g) Serve as the point of contact for HIPAA Privacy and Security compliance, monitoring and assuring staff compliance with HIPAA training requirements. The officer will administrate the databases that track data disclosures and complaints; conduct Privacy and Security risk assessments; participate in the HIPAA compliance quality assurance and improvement process; and report findings to the CG P/SO.

(h) Serves as the local P/SO for the HSWL Directorate.

(i) Clinics shall be evaluated on their privacy data protection as part of their triennial HPAP survey with results included in the final HPAP report. Clinics will also be evaluated on a periodic basis to ensure they have adequate administrative and physical security. Records must be protected from viewing or inadvertent exposure by storing them in cabinets or other containers that, when unattended, are locked.

c. Local HSWL clinic Privacy and Security Officers.

(1) Each HSWL clinic P/SO will serve as the point of contact for their assigned treatment facility. The HSWL clinic P/SO oversees activities related to the implementation and maintenance of local clinic HIPAA SOPs covering the access to and privacy of patient health information.

(2) Health Services Administrators are responsible for designating in writing the clinic's HIPAA P/SO. A copy of this letter of designation shall be forwarded to the HSWL-SC P/SO. Whenever there is a change in the clinic's P/SO, the Health Services Administrator must designate another member as P/SO and notify the HSWL-SC P/SO of the change and provide a copy of the designation letter within 10 working days of the effective date of such letter.

(3) Responsibilities of the HSWL clinic P/SO are:

(a) Oversee, direct, monitor and ensure delivery of initial HIPAA privacy and security training and orientation to all clinical staff. Ensure annual refresher training is conducted in order to maintain workforce awareness and to introduce any changes to HIPAA privacy or security policies to the health care workforce. The P/SO may share or delegate responsibilities for monitoring compliance with HIPAA training requirements to another appropriately trained health care workforce individual as a HIPAA Training Administrator at the unit.

(b) Perform initial and periodic information privacy and security risk assessments and conduct related ongoing compliance monitoring activities in coordination with applicable CG Directives. Report findings as required.

(c) Ensure a mechanism is in place within all respective treatment facilities for receiving, documenting, tracking, investigating all complaints concerning the organization's privacy and security policies and procedures in coordination and collaboration with other similar functions, and, when necessary, legal counsel.

(d) Document disclosures of Protected Health Information (PHI).

(e) Understand the content of health information in its clinical, research and business context.

(f) Understand the decision-making processes that rely on health information. Identify and monitor the flow of information within the clinic and throughout the local health care network.

    (g) Serve as privacy/security liaison for users of clinical and administrative systems.

    (h) Collaborate with other health care professionals to ensure appropriate security measures are in place to safeguard protected health information and to facilitate exchange of information between entities.

    (i) Initiate, facilitate and promote activities to foster information privacy awareness within the organization and related entities.

    (j) Serve as the advocate for the patient relative to the confidentiality and privacy of health information.

    (k) Conduct an annual internal assessment regarding its processes and procedures for the protection of PII and PHI and develop a contingency plan for the inadvertent release of PII and PHI.

    (l) Ensure adequate health record security provisions are required for the protection of PHI contained in Coast Guard health records, including electronic files.

3. Permitted Uses and Disclosures for Treatment, Payment, and Operations. The USCG Health Care Program is generally permitted to use or disclose, without patient authorization, protected health information for purposes of treatment, payment, or healthcare operations (TPO). Any questions regarding use and disclosures for purposes of TPO can be directed to the CG HIPAA P/SO.

4. Uses and Disclosures for which an Authorization is Required.

    a. Patient authorization is generally required for any use or disclosure of protected health information that falls outside the definition of TPO, or otherwise permitted by the HIPAA Privacy Rule.

    b. The CG Health Care Program may not condition treatment, payment, or benefits eligibility on an individual granting an authorization, except in limited circumstances.

    c. Authorization for Disclosure of Medical or Dental Information, Form DD-2870 fulfills the requirements for authorizing PHI.

5. Minimum Necessary Rule. The HIPAA 'Minimum Necessary' Rule is defined as the minimum amount of PHI that is reasonably needed to achieve the purpose of a requested use, disclosure or request for PHI.

    a. All elements of the CG Health Care program must make reasonable efforts to limit its use, disclosure of, and requests for PHI to the minimum necessary in order to accomplish the intended purpose of the use, disclosure, or request. This includes making a reasonable effort to limit access to PHI to those in its workforce who need access based on their role in the organization.

    b. The minimum necessary rule does not apply to:

        (1) Uses, disclosures to, or requests by a healthcare provider for treatment purposes.

        (2) Uses or disclosures made to the individual (patient).

(3) Uses or disclosures that are authorized by the individual pursuant to a valid authorization, signed by the patient or a personal representative, so long as the uses or disclosures are consistent with the authorization.

(4) Uses or disclosures that are required by state or other law, statutes, and regulations (unless prohibited by the Privacy Act of 1974).

(5) Uses or disclosures for purposes of training medical residents, medical students, nursing students and other medical trainees as part of their medical training program. If required, the entire medical record may be requested and/or disclosed for training purposes.

(6) Uses or disclosures which are required to comply with standard Health Insurance Portability and Accountability Act (HIPAA) transactions (however, the minimum necessary standard applies to the "optional" data elements which may be included in these transactions) or other HIPAA Administrative Simplification Regulations.

(7) Disclosures to the Secretary of Health and Human Services (HHS) required under HIPAA for enforcement purposes.

6. Individual Privacy Rights Related to Protected Health Information.

   a. All CG clinics will ensure that beneficiaries who encounter the facility receive a Notice of Privacy Practices (NoPP).

   b. Patients have the right to inspect and obtain a copy of their PHI. A CG clinic may deny a patient's request for access under any of the following conditions:

      (1) The PHI is psychotherapy notes;

      (2) Information is compiled for use in a civil, criminal, or administrative action or proceeding;

      (3) The PHI is subject to the Clinical Laboratory Improvements Amendments (CLIA) of 1988 to the extent that access to the individual is prohibited by law;

      (4) The PHI contains quality assurance information; or,

      (5) Any PHI that was provided from a source other than a health care provider under a promise of confidentiality.

   c. In certain situations, a patient may request that the medical facility amend or supplement their PHI. Requests may be denied if the PHI is or was not:

      (1) Created by the medical clinic;

      (2) Part of a designated record set; and,

      (3) Available for inspection.

7. PHI Disclosure and the Military Mission.

   a. The implementation of the HIPAA Privacy Rule shall not compromise the provision of quality healthcare or the military mission. 45 CFR 164.512 states

b. that "a covered entity may use and disclose PHI of individuals who are Armed Forces personnel for activities deemed necessary by appropriate military command authorities to assure the proper execution of the military mission."

c. Appropriate Military Command Authorities include the following:

   (1) All Commanders who exercise authority (in the individual's chain of command) over an individual who is a member of the Armed Forces, or other person designated by such a Commander to receive PHI in order to carry out an activity under the authority of the Commander.

   (2) The Secretary of Homeland Security when the Coast Guard is not operating as a service in the Department of the Navy.

   (3) Any official delegated authority by the Secretary of Homeland Security to take an action designed to ensure the proper execution of the military mission.

d. Activities or Purposes that Qualify under this Stipulation:

   (1) To determine the member's fitness for duty, including but not limited to the member's compliance with standards and all activities carried out under the authority of Coast Guard Weight and Body Fat Standards Program Manual, COMDTINST M1020.8 (series), Coast Guard Medical Manual, COMDTINST M6000.1(series), Coast Guard Aviation Medicine Manual, COMDTINST M6410.3 (series), Physical Disabilities Evaluation System, COMDTINST M1850.2 (series), Periodic Health Assessment, COMDTINST 6150.3 (series), and similar requirements.

   (2) To determine the member's fitness to perform any particular mission, assignment, order, or duty, including compliance with any actions required as a precondition to performance of such mission, assignment, order, or duty.

   (3) To carry out activities under the authority of Chapter 12 in this Manual and the Department of Defense Directive 6490.2, Joint Medical Surveillance.

   (4) To report on casualties in any military operation or activity in accordance with applicable military regulations or procedures.

   (5) To carry out any other activity necessary to the proper execution of the mission of the Armed Forces.

e. Accounting for Disclosures to Command Authorities: Coast Guard clinics are required to account for disclosures made to command authorities. If the member of the Armed Forces voluntarily gives his health information to a command authority, this is not an accountable disclosure and therefore the clinic is not required to account for it.

8. Accounting for Disclosures.

   a. By law the CG must be able to provide an accounting of those disclosures to a patient upon request.

      (1) CG medical facilities must maintain a history of when and to whom

disclosures of PHI are made for purposes other than treatment, payment and healthcare operations (TPO).

(2) Authorizations and restrictions from an individual are included in the information that is required for tracking purposes. The HIPAA Rule suggests that disclosures for the purpose of appointment reminders, such as for upcoming, missed, or cancelled appointments, can be treated as disclosures for purposes of treatment.

b. An individual has a right to receive an accounting of disclosures of PHI made in the 6 years prior to the date that the accounting is requested. An accounting of disclosures is not needed for the following:

(1) To carry out treatment, payment and healthcare operations;

(2) To individuals or their personal representative of PHI about them, (e.g. individual provides his/her command with a duty status chit or up/down chit Medical Recommendation for Flying Duty, Form CG-6020);

(3) When a signed authorization form (such as a Authorization for Disclosure or Medical or Dental Information, Form DD-2870) allows for the disclosure;

(4) For the facility's directory, to persons involved in the individual's care, for disaster relief or other notification purposes;

(5) For national security or intelligence purposes, such as disclosures to the Security Center (SECCEN);

(6) To correctional institutions or law enforcement officials; or,

(7) As part of a limited data set.

c. The accounting for each disclosure shall include:

(1) The date of the disclosure;

(2) The name of the entity or person who received the PHI and, if known, the address of such entity or person;

(3) A brief description of the PHI disclosed;

(4) A brief statement of the purpose of the disclosure that reasonably informs the individual of the basis for the disclosure.

d. A single accounting of disclosure is permitted, if multiple disclosures of PHI to the same person or entity are made for a single purpose. This single accounting may be utilized only for disclosures that occur on a set periodic basis such as medical boards or binnacle lists containing PHI to a commander or the commander's designee(s). The disclosure accounting must include:

(1) All the elements as outlined in Paragraph 8-c.

(2) The frequency, periodicity, or number of the disclosures made during the accounting period.

(3) The date of the last such disclosure during the accounting period.

e. To comply with the requirements for disclosures, the **DHA** provides the Protected Health Information Management Tool (PHIMT), an electronic disclosure-tracking database. The PHIMT stores information about all disclosures, authorizations, and restrictions that are made for a particular patient. PHIMT has a functionality built into it that can provide an accounting of disclosures, if necessary.

f. A CG clinic must provide an accounting of disclosures within sixty days of the request. If the clinic cannot honor an accounting of disclosures within the sixty day period, it must provide information to the requestor as to the reason for the delay and expected completion date. The clinic may extend the time to provide the accounting by no more than thirty days. Only one extension is permitted per request.

9. <u>Breaches and Unauthorized Uses and Disclosures of Protected Health Information</u>.

a. The term 'breach' generally means the unauthorized acquisition, access, use, or disclosure of protected health information which compromises the security or privacy of such information. There are three exceptions to the definition of "breach":

(1) The first exception applies to the unintentional acquisition, access, or use of protected health information by a workforce member acting under the authority of a covered entity or business associate.

(2) The second exception applies to the inadvertent disclosure of protected health information from a person authorized to access protected health information at a covered entity or business associate to another person authorized to access protected health information at the covered entity or business associate. In both cases, the information cannot be further used or disclosed in a manner not permitted by the Privacy Rule.

(3) The final exception to breach applies if the covered entity or business associate has a good faith belief that the unauthorized individual, to whom the impermissible disclosure was made, would not have been able to retain the information

b. If anyone within the CG discovers evidence or circumstances which would suggest that a breach of security of a system containing protected health information (PHI) or of an unintentional disclosure of PHI may have occurred, the Health Services Administrator and HSWL clinic P/SO shall be immediately notified.

c. Procedures of the HSWL clinic P/SO:

(1) Notify the HSWL-SC P/SO and CG P/SO via email or telephonically. The CG P/SO can provide further guidance on breach response procedures and will notify and communicate with the **DHA** Privacy Office, as necessary.

(2) Privacy Incident Response, Notification, and Reporting Procedures for Personally Identifiable Information (PII), COMDTINST 5260.5 (series) shall be followed, to include submitting a Privacy Incident Report, Form CG-5260A to the TIS-SG-CGCIRT.

(3) Receive, document, and initiate an investigation of the incident, including conducting interviews of all individuals knowledgeable of the circumstances of the incident, or of the technical systems or administrative procedures which may have lead created the vulnerability.

d. Time line. The HSWL clinic P/SO through the local command authority shall provide notification of all individuals whose PHI may have been compromised within 10 business days of the conclusion of the investigation of the incident. This notification shall identify or outline:

(1) The nature and scope of the incident and the circumstances surrounding the loss, theft, compromise or disclosure of the PHI;

(2) Specific data that was involved;

(3) Actions taken by the local facility to remedy the vulnerability;

(4) Potential risks incurred by the affected individuals as a result of the disclosure, compromise, loss or theft of PHI;

(5) Actions which the individuals can take to protect against potential harm; and,

(6) Resources for obtaining further information and/or a point of contact to address any further questions the individual may have related to the potential compromise of PHI.

e. Final report. The HSWL clinic P/SO will submit to the HSWL-SC P/SO and CG P/SO a final report containing a description of the findings of the investigation, efforts made to mitigate any harm resulting from the disclosure, and corrective actions take to remedy weakness of technical systems, or administrative policies or procedures which lead to the vulnerability.

f. Lessons learned. The HSWL-SC P/SO will disseminate lessons learned from the incident to all HSWL clinics P/SOs and appropriate command authorities so that local systems, policies and procedures can be review and appropriate corrective action and/or training can be completed.

10. Responding to HIPAA Complaints.

a. Beneficiaries may file complaints regarding perceived misuse or disclosure of their PHI. This information includes demographics such as age, address, or e-mail, and relates to past, present or future health information and related health care services.

b. It is encouraged that complaints be addressed locally or at the lowest possible level. However, inquiries or complaints may be received at any level of the CG Health Care Program or at **DHA**. Individuals also have the right to make inquiries or address complaints directly to the Department of Health and

Chapter 13. G. Page 9

CH-1

Human Services (HHS), HHS Office for Civil Rights (OCR) web site gives instructions to individuals who wish to make a HIPAA complaint.

(1) Beneficiary complaints should be directed in writing to the local HSWL clinic P/SO. The complaint must include:

   (a) Beneficiary's name, address, phone number, and clinic accessed for care;

   (b) Date complaint taken/submitted;

   (c) Description of complaint and approximate date incident occurred; and,

   (d) Facility and location where incident occurred.

(2) The HSWL clinic P/SO shall notify the HSWL-SC P/SO and CG P/SO of all complaints, so that the CG P/SO can provide assistance and guidance as necessary.

(3) The HSWL clinic P/SO is responsible for determining whether a complaint is a valid HIPAA complaint, a grievance under another privacy law, or not a HIPAA complaint. The CG P/SO will be available to assist and advise as needed.

(4) To the extent necessary, the local HSWL clinic P/SO will investigate the incident and interview witnesses, managers and staff. The scene of the incident can be visited, action can be taken to limit scope of incident, and copies of relevant files should be retrieved. Disclosures may be identified as incidental to routine business, accidental or due to malicious intent.

(5) The HSWL clinic P/SO will prepare a summary of findings and forward to the HSWL-SC P/SO and CG P/SO for review and endorsement.

(6) The complaining party must receive a written response in a timely manner. The designated review authority (P/SO) shall reply within 30 days of the date of receipt of the complaint. If additional review is necessary, the reviewer can request an extension for an additional 30 days. When this occurs, the individual must be notified in writing that the issue is under investigation and the extension is being put into effect. In the case of complaints made by beneficiaries directly to the HHS and forwarded to **DHA** for resolution, responses are required to be provided to the CG P/SO who will review and forward to the **DHA** Privacy Office for review and endorsement to HHS. Direct communication to the complaining beneficiary will be at the discretion of HHS.

(7) Written documentation of the complaint and its disposition must be maintained by the activity receiving the inquiry or complaint. Each clinic is required to ensure appropriate documentation. Documentation must be maintained for a minimum of six years from the submission of the complaint.

c. Additional Procedures for HIPAA Complaints Determined to be PHI Breaches.

(1) If the complaint is determined to be a breach of PHI, procedures included in Paragraph 9, c-f will be followed.

(2) The CG P/SO will review and submit all required documentation to the **DHA** Privacy Office for review and endorsement.

d. Complaints Received at Commands Other Than Treatment Facilities.

(1) Whenever possible, complaints received at Commands other than CG treatment facilities, should be redirected to the appropriate local HSWL clinic P/SO for investigation and response.

(2) Commands shall notify the HSWL-SC P/SO and CG P/SO Commandant (CG-1122) by email of all other complaints. The HSWL-SC P/SO and/or CG P/SO will assist and advise the Command's investigating officer; coordinate the response with legal counsel, where necessary; and review the written response of the investigating officer. If necessary, the CG P/SO will coordinate the response with the **DHA** Privacy Office.

11. Electronic Transmission of Protected Health Information.

a. Coast Guard Messaging System. Messages should not contain personally identifiable health information. This includes listing the name of the individual and any disease code (i.e., International Classification of Disease (ICD-9 or ICD-10) or Common Procedural Terminology (CPT)) which be used to identify the disease or condition of the individual. Messages requiring transmission of personally identifiable health information shall use the Inpatient Hospitalization Message format (see Paragraph. b below).

b. Inpatient Hospitalization Messages. Protected Health Information (PHI) will be sent utilizing the procedure described in Chapter 7.B.(3)(b) for the Disease Alert Report or Chapter 2.A.(2)(b) utilizing the Inpatient Hospitalization system. Send only the minimum necessary information to accomplish the intended purpose of the use, disclosure or request via e-mail to HQS-DG-HSWL Inpatient Hospitalization, as appropriate. This e-mail will only be viewed by limited command designated individuals at HQ and HSWL-SC with a need to know. No other individuals shall be included or copied on this e-mail, nor shall the e-mail containing PHI be forwarded after the fact.

c. Faxing Protected Health Information. Any individual who has access to protected health information (PHI) in the course of their duties is obligated to maintain the security of that information. Best practices to maintain the security of PHI include only faxing PHI to secure faxes, in other words, faxes in secured spaces where only those who utilize PHI have access to the secure fax. If information is sent to any other non-secure fax, it is required that the sender alert the receiver to stand by and receive the fax so that the fax containing PHI cannot be inadvertently intercepted by someone without authorization to receive and use PHI. The receiver should then contact the sender to acknowledge safe receipt of the fax containing PHI.

d. Recommended Disclaimer on Protected Health Information Sent Electronically. The following disclaimer statement is recommended by the **DHA** Privacy Office. It may be placed in the footer of a Fax Cover Sheet for the transmission of PHI or may be used at the end of an email containing PHI. The word "Confidential" in bold should be placed at the beginning of the footer above this disclaimer as depicted below:

CONFIDENTIAL

This document may contain information covered under the Privacy Act, 5 USC552(a), and/or the Health Insurance Portability and Accountability Act (PL 104-191) and its various implementing regulations and must be protected in accordance with those provisions. Healthcare information is personal and sensitive and must be treated accordingly. If this correspondence contains healthcare information it is being provided to you after appropriate authorization from the patient or under circumstances that don't require patient authorization. You, the recipient, are obligated to maintain it in a safe, secure and confidential manner. Redisclosure without additional patient consent or as permitted by law is prohibited. Unauthorized redisclosure or failure to maintain confidentiality subjects you to application of appropriate sanction. If you have received this correspondence in error, please notify the sender at once and destroy any copies you have made.

12. <u>HIPAA Training Requirements</u>.

   a. <u>45 Code of Federal Regulations (CFR)</u>. 45 CFR 164.530 (b) specifies the training requirement standards under HIPAA. All CG health care workforce members are required to complete designated training within 30 working days of reporting on duty to the CG or being assigned to a specific CG unit. Meeting with the local HSWL clinic Privacy and Security Official should be included as a required element of all in-processing for health care workforce members.

      (1) The HSWL clinic P/SO will provide the individual with the domain identification number for their respective unit to complete web-based training requirements. When a health care workforce member leaves the treatment facility, the clinic P/SO should direct the member to change the domain identifier to that of the receiving treatment facility where the member will be assigned.

      (2) Required training includes at least (1) those courses corresponding to the appropriate HIPAA Job Position provided through the **DoD Joint Knowledge Online (JKO) website**; (2) training on the clinic's policies and procedures; (3) any other HIPAA privacy and security training as determined by the HSWL clinic P/SO.

      (3) Training shall be completed by utilizing the web-based training courses available through the **DoD JKO site** http://jko.jten.mil.

      (4) **These requirements apply to all active duty and reserve members, contract staff and Auxiliarists within the CG health care workforce.**

      (5) **Completion of the HIPAA core and refresher training courses is required prior to obtaining access and for continued access to paper and electronic health records.**

(6) CG health care workforce members are required to complete the HIPAA refresher training annually. It is highly recommended that they complete the training during their birth month, but it is at the discretion of their respective Regional Manager and/or Clinic Administrator, who are also responsible for tracking completion of training.

13. Other CG Members Who Utilize Protected Health Information.

(a) Other members of the CG may routinely or occasionally have access to or utilize protected health information in the course of their duties. Although these members are not considered part of the "health care workforce," and therefore, are not required by law and implementing regulations (see 45 CFR 164.530 (b)) to complete HIPAA training, it is critical that these members are aware of the intent of HIPAA and maintain the privacy and confidentiality of protected health information with which they are entrusted. To accomplish this objective, members assigned to the following organizations or performing duties in the following roles should complete appropriate HIPAA training:

(1) National Maritime Center;

(2) CG Personnel Command/Physical Disabilities Evaluation Board;

(3) Special Needs Program staff;

(4) Command Drug and Alcohol Representatives/ Drug and Alcohol Program staff; and,

(5) Others as deemed necessary by the CG P/SO and/or **COs.**

H. Quality Improvement Studies.

1. Background. In the early 1990s the CG established a Monitoring and Evaluation (M&E) program to examine areas of clinical care the CG deemed important in order to assess how well clinics provided this care. The M&E program centered on the review of historical data and, thus, was a retroactive program. Further, the program was strictly a QA program in that it was designed to ensure a set standard of care was met in specific areas. M&Es did not necessarily seek to improve care beyond a set standard. Quality Improvement Studies (QISs) will replace M&Es as the primary tool for evaluating healthcare delivery in clinics. M&Es will no longer be used as a QA tool. QISs provide a framework so that current QA clinic standards of care themselves are reviewed for improvement. Further, QISs are proactive versus retroactive in nature because data from QISs are reviewed as they become available.

2. Responsibilities.

   a. HSWL SC. Monitors the QIS Program activities. The HSWL SC provides guidance to the program.

   b. Quality Improvement Coordinator. The QI Coordinator ensures that at least four QISs are completed annually, in a timely manner, and in the proper format and are documented in the QI Focus Group (QIFG) meeting minutes. The QI Coordinator ensures that delegated tasks are completed by the appropriate clinic personnel.

   c. Quality Improvement Focus Group. The QIFG meets at least quarterly and is responsible for approving and monitoring the QISs conducted in the clinic. The QIFG provides guidance to QIS investigators and other members of the staff involved in implementing QISs. On-going QISs are discussed in QIFG meetings and documented in its minutes. The QIFG, which includes providers and administrators, participates in the resolution of the problem or issue identified.

   d. Clinic personnel. Ensure important problems that address clinical, administrative or cost issues, and patient outcomes are brought before the QIFG to initiate as QISs. All personnel participate in the identification and resolution of problems.

3. Definitions.

   a. Problem. Any question to be considered, resolved, or answered in order to meet or improve upon Accreditation Association if Ambulatory Health Care (AAAHC) or Chapter 13 of this Manual.

   b. Quality Improvement Study. In a healthcare setting, a tool used to systematically review a single problem of healthcare delivery or operations within a clinic in order to determine if there is an improved and sustainable solution to the problem.

   c. Quality Assurance, Quality Improvement. See Chapter 13-A-8 for the definitions of Quality Assurance and Quality Improvement.

4. <u>General Information</u>. The QIS Program must be active (implements at least 4 studies per year), organized (utilizes a systematic, "closed loop" process), peer-based (results reviewed by the QIFG, documented in the QIFG minutes, posted in clinic public folder for HSWL SC review), and integrated (includes issues from all clinical and administrative departments within the clinic, incorporates results into the clinic standard operating procedures, and provides staff training when necessary).

5. <u>QIS Focus</u>. QISs address or identify issues including standards of care, quality of care delivered, effectiveness of healthcare delivery, efficiency of operations, and additional issues or concerns unique to individual clinics. The QIS process must focus on one problem or issue per study although the clinic may conduct more than one QIS concurrently.

6. <u>QIS Process</u>. The QIS process is a sequential process that roughly parallels the scientific method. The process is outlined in a flow-sheet (See Figure 13-H-1).

    a. Step 1: Identify problem.

    b. Step 2: Gather information on problem.

    c. Step 3: Develop solution to problem.

    d. Step 4: Conduct training on solution.

    e. Step 5: Implement solution to problem.

    f. Step 6: Report results of implemented solution.

    g. Step 7: Evaluate solution to problem.

7. <u>QIS Report Form</u>. Clinic QI activities are reported on the Quality Improvement Study Report Template, Form CG-6000-6 which follows the stepwise QIS process.

8. <u>Frequency of Quality Improvement Studies</u>. Quality improvement is a continuous process therefore clinics must initiate a minimum of four QISs per calendar year. QISs should be spread throughout the year when possible and involve different clinical areas when possible (e.g. lab, pharmacy, medical, administration).

9. <u>Completing the QIS Report Form</u>.

    a. <u>Overview</u>. The QIS Report form is a major component of implementing a successful QI program. It serves as the building block for QI interventions and a record of QI activities. This section describes the major components of the form and how to complete it.

    b. <u>Name of study</u>. Concise yet descriptive such as "health record tracking," "lab results monitoring," or "prescription error rate."

    c. <u>Investigator</u>. The person responsible for completing the QIS and presenting its findings to the QIFG.

    d. <u>Study</u>. Select if the QIS is an initial study or a follow-up study.

e. Date completed. The date on which the current QIS Report form was completed.

f. Problem Statement. The specific problem is described in one or two sentences. The name of the study should reflect what the problem is. Each QIS addresses a single problem. Each QIS must only address one problem. If there are multiple problems, a QIS must be done for each one.

g. Background to problem/Known facts of problem. The background to the problem is described and the known facts of the problem are listed (who, what, when, where, how). Information on the problem is evaluated for reliability.

h. Parameters of problem. The parameters that define the problem are determined. Problems with greater negative consequences that occur frequently should take precedence over those with lesser consequences that occur less frequently.

i. Area of Care. Select the area of care that best describes the nature of the problem:

   (1) Administrative. Examples include health record completeness, record tracking system, referral tracking, staffing utilization, staff satisfaction, medical/legal issues, cost issues, patient flow, health readiness, quality controls in clinic departments, monitoring of care, assessing patient satisfaction, wasteful practices, and access to care.

   (2) Ancillary. Examples include monitoring abnormal results, radiograph retakes.

   (3) Clinical. Examples include tracking management of contagious disease cases, assessing for appropriateness of care according to standard guidelines, assessing changes in outcomes based on changes in practice, medications or ancillary treatments.

   (4) Dental. Examples include annual Type 2 exam process, ensuring proper sterilization of instruments, and endodontic and periodontal treatment follow-up.

   (5) Medical. Examples include physical exam process, diagnostic testing procedures, practice patterns of providers, and comparisons to national standards of care.

   (6) Patient outcome. Examples include adverse events, medication errors, deviation from standard of care, clinical procedure processes, and peer review findings.

   (7) Pharmaceutical. Examples include Non-Formulary Medication Utilization, Appropriate Use of Antibiotics to treat URIs, and Improving Patient Medication Outcomes.

j. <u>Parameters of problem Consequence</u>. Determine what happens if solution to problem is not found. This step may assist clinics to determine on which issues to focus their efforts.

    (1) <u>Devastating</u>. Problem results in intolerable outcome, loss of life, injury, economic penalty or legal issues.

    (2) <u>Serious</u>. Problem could result in injury, hazard or economic penalty.

    (3) <u>Moderate</u>. Problem will probably not cause hazard or economic penalty.

    (4) <u>Low</u>. Problem does not have much implication to health or economics.

k. <u>Standards used to evaluate problem</u>. This element usually applies to clinical QISs that involve the comparison of clinic standards of care against national treatment or practice guidelines. Complete if applicable.

l. <u>Proposed solution to problem</u>. Describe how and what information was gathered to determine course of action. Describe specifically what steps the clinic will take to address the problem. This will take a paragraph to describe.

m. <u>Desired outcome of solution</u>. Discuss specifically what the clinic hopes to attain by implementation of the solution.

n. <u>Training Date</u>. Give date on which the staff was trained on the proposed solution to the problem. Must ensure staff is trained so they know how to implement the solution and what is expected of them.

o. <u>Training Aids</u>. Check applicable boxes. Generally, solutions that involve tasks with higher levels of consequence if an error occurs or those that involve tasks that occur less frequently require greater training intervention than those that have less consequences or occur more frequently. The QIFG must determine what training strategies to use in order to successfully implement the corrective solution. Training must involve at least two strategies that include memory tools, lectures, checklists, flow charts and practice/rehearsal.

p. <u>Implement solution to problem</u>. Each task must have a person assigned to it who is responsible for its completion by a specified date. These tasks include those that originate from the statements listed under "proposed solution to problem." Tasks are implemented concurrently or sequentially depending on the problem. As each task is completed the date is noted in the "completion date" column. The responsible party does not have to be the investigator. Progress is reported in the meeting minutes of the QIFG. The QIFG determines if the results achieved by the intervention provide sustainable improvements. If the solution involves a long-term project (i.e. one over six months to implement or review) such as an area renovation, check the appropriate box noting this fact. Interpret the QIS Flowchart in light of the time adjustments required for long-term projects.

q. <u>Report results of the implemented solution</u>. Complete the "Initial QIS" section for the first study, the "Follow-up QIS" section for the second study and the "Additional QIS" section if a third study is warranted. For long term projects note the appropriate follow-up dates in the text.

r. Evaluate solution to problem: Initial QIS. Check whether the solution was sustained or not sustained and fill-in the appropriate boxes. Note when the findings were documented in the QIFG meeting minutes.

s. Evaluate solution to problem: Follow-up QIS. Check whether the solution was sustained or not sustained after the follow-up study was concluded. If sustained, check the appropriate boxes for what actions were taken to integrate the solution into clinic operations. Check what training tools were used to educate staff on new proposed solution. Note when the findings were documented in the QIFG meeting minutes.

t. Evaluate solution to problem: Additional QIS (if needed). For QISs that involve areas of high risk to patients or could result in devastating consequences if not resolved, an additional evaluation may be desired. Check whether the solution was sustained or not sustained after the additional study was initiated. Check what training tools were used to educate staff on new proposed solution. A new QIS Report Form must be started if the implemented solution is not sustained after a third study. Note when the findings were documented in the QIFG meeting minutes.

u. Evaluate solution to problem: HSWL SC assistance.

10. Follow-up Reporting. The QIS Report Form is designed to be used for the initial and follow-up study (or studies) for a particular problem. For follow-up or additional QISs add the findings to the "Report Results of Implemented Solution" section. Results are recorded in the QIFG minutes.

11. Integration. Once a follow-up or additional QIS results in a sustainable solution, the corrective solution must be incorporated into the SOP and results reported in the QIFG minutes.

12. Filing. The HSWL SC will establish a filing process for the clinics such as public folders or microsite on CG Central to ensure sharing of information.

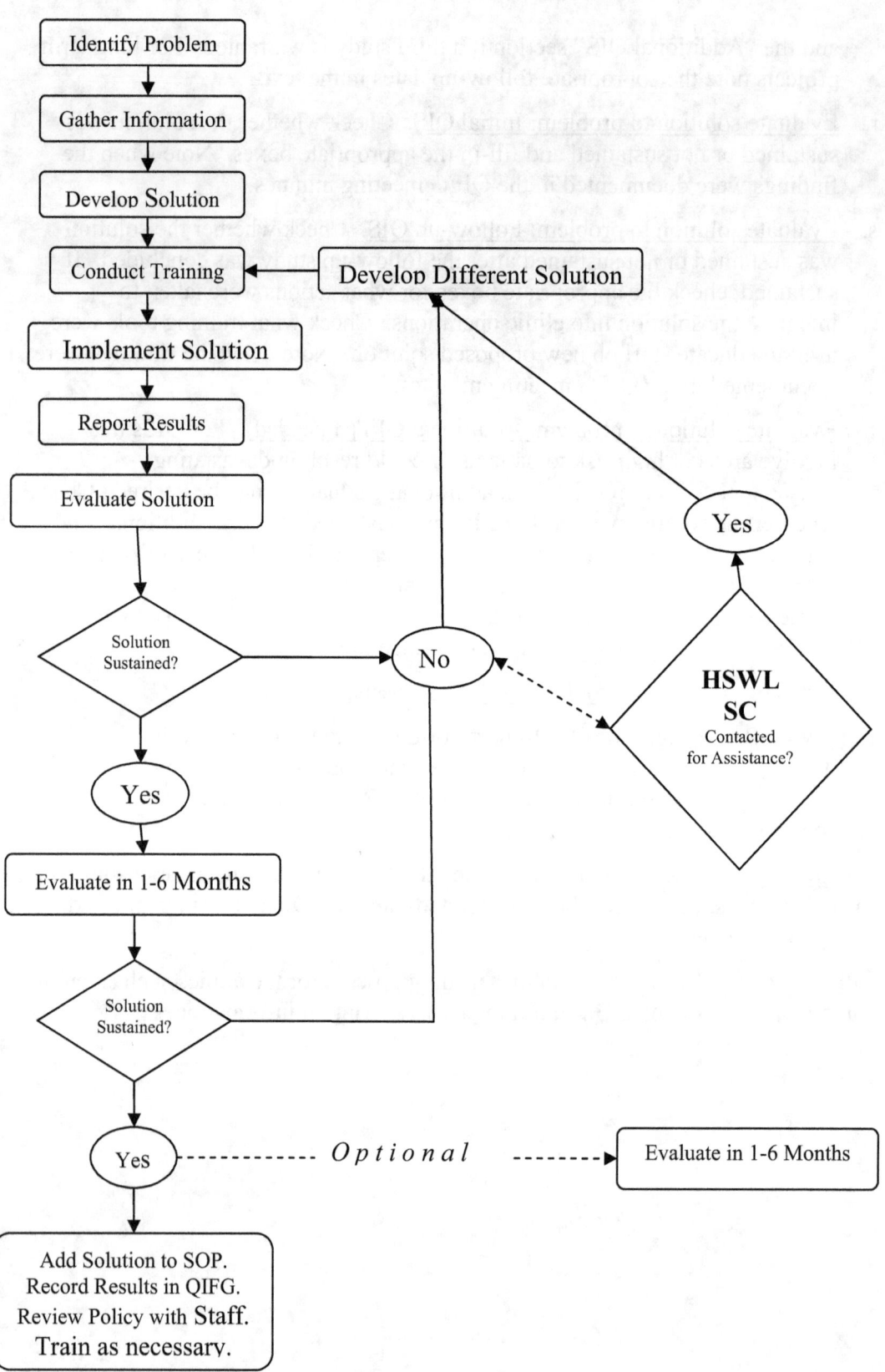

I. Peer Review Program.

1. Purpose. In striving to improve the quality of care and promote more effective and efficient utilization of facilities and services, an accredited organization maintains an active, integrated, organized, peer-based program of quality management and improvement that links peer review, quality improvement activities, and risk management in an organized, systematic way.

2. Characteristics of a Peer Review Program. The CG peer review program maintains an active and organized process for peer review that is integrated into the quality management and improvement program, evidenced by the following characteristics.

    a. Health care providers. Health care providers understand, support and participate in a peer review program through organized mechanisms and are responsible to the governing body. The peer review activities are evidenced in the quality improvement program. Health care providers participate in the development and application of the criteria used to evaluate the care they provide.

    b. Commandant (CG-1122). Commandant (CG-1122) provides ongoing monitoring of important aspects of the care provided by physicians, dentists, mid-level providers, and other health care professionals. Monitoring important aspects of care by individual practitioners is necessary for monitoring individual performance and establishing internal benchmarks.

    c. Data criteria. Data related to established criteria are collected in an on-going manner and periodically evaluated to identify acceptable or unacceptable trends or occurrences that affect patient outcome.

    d. Clinical privileges. Results of peer review activities are used as part of the process for granting continuation of clinical privileges.

    e. Results of Reviews. Peer review activities are not designed to be punitive in nature, but can be used to identify trends requiring improvements, to enhance or improve professional competence, skill, and quality of performance of health care providers, and to guide educational programs and activities consistent with the CG mission, goals, and objectives.

3. Definitions.

    a. Current Procedural Terminology (CPT). The CPT is an acronym for Current Procedural Terminology. CPT codes are published by the American Medical Association, and the fourth edition, the most current, is used. The purpose of the coding system is to provide uniform language that accurately describes medical, surgical, and diagnostic services.

    b. International Classification of Diseases, 9th Revision, Clinical Modification (ICD-9-CM). The ICD-9-CM coding system is used to code signs, symptoms, injuries, diseases, and conditions.

c. Code on Dental Procedures and Nomenclature (CDT). CDT is an acronym for Code on Dental Procedures and Nomenclature. The American Dental Association's (ADA) Code on Dental Procedures and Nomenclature (CDT) is used to record and report dental procedures. It is the dental equivalent of Current Procedure Terminology (CPT) codes for other-than-dental procedures. Hence the ADA's choice of the official abbreviation CDT rather than CDPN.

d. Benchmarking. A systematic comparison of products, services, or work processes of similar organizations, departments or practitioners to identify best practices known to date for the purpose of continuous quality improvement.

4. Responsibilities.

a. Commandant (CG-112). Establish and maintain contract with an electronic peer review data collection and organization database, known as Medical Encounter Review System (MERS).

b. HSWL SC. Conduct second level review, if necessary, based on report from the CG Professional Review Committee (PRC) and address (through the Regional Practice) any significant treads identified to improve quality of care.

5. Process.

a. Review of Providers. All coast guard providers actively engaged in patient care are required to participate in peer review through MERS. At the beginning of each month, 5 encounters will be randomly selected from the previous month's encounters and assigned to randomly selected individual providers with commensurate credentials/qualifications for review. Each reviewer will receive an e-mail notification and has 30 days to complete the assigned peer reviews online. After 30 days, incomplete reviews are reported by the system to the reviewer's immediate supervisor and made available to the HSWL SC chain of command.

b. Mid Level Review. All Coast Guard physicians who supervise mid-level providers are required to use MERS for their supervisory review of mid-level providers. Supervisors will be assigned 5 encounters for review for each mid-level provider every month. The supervisor has 30 days to complete the assigned reviews. After 30 days, incomplete reviews will be reported by the system to the Senior Medical Executive and made available to the HSWL SC chain of command.

c. Personal Peer Review Scores. All providers are required to review their personal peer review scores monthly in MERS in order to complete the feedback loop. This is accomplished by checking the box at the end of each peer review score report.

d. <u>Commandant (CG-1122)</u>. Commandant (CG-1122) will use data provided from the reports to track enterprise-wide trends and establish benchmarks for improvement.

e. <u>Findings</u>. Findings determined to warrant a second review will be conducted by HSWL SC per guidance from Commandant (CG-1122).

J. Infection Control Program (Exposure Control Plan).

1. Introduction.

a. Standard Precautions. Identifying potentially infectious patients by medical history, physical examination, or readily available laboratory tests is not always possible. Extended periods often exist between the time a person becomes infected with a microbial agent and the time when laboratory tests can detect the associated antigens or antibodies. Consequently, even if a patient tests negative, he or she may still be infectious. Health care personnel must assume that all blood/body fluids and contaminated instruments and materials are infectious and routinely use Standard Precautions to protect themselves and patients.

b. Safety Procedures. All procedures should be available to minimize the sources and transmission of infections, including adequate surveillance techniques.

c. Protection. All CG systems must provide for the protection of patients, staff and the environment.

d. Exposure. While CG health services personnel and emergency medical technicians must be seriously concerned with the risk of exposure to human immunodeficiency virus (HIV), the risk of contracting other infectious diseases, such as Hepatitis B virus (HBV), is much greater. HBV infection can result in serious physical debilitation and adversely affect a practitioner's ability to provide health care. Once infected, a person also poses a potential risk to future patients as an HBV infection "carrier." Infection control practices that prevent HBV transmission also prevent HIV transmission. Since 1982 a safe, effective vaccine to prevent Hepatitis B has been available; it stimulates active immunity against HBV infection and provides over 90% protection against the virus for 7 or more years after vaccination.

e. Occupational Safety and Health Administration (OSHA). The OSHA Blood borne Pathogens (BBP) Standard requires the use of Standard Precautions to protect the healthcare worker from exposure to bloodborne pathogens. The basic principle of Standard Precautions is the assumption that all patients are potentially infectious. Therefore, the risk of exposure to blood or other potentially infectious materials (OPIM) posed by a procedure dictates the level of precautions, rather than the perceived infectivity of the patient. In 1996, the Hospital Infection Control Practices Advisory Committee (HICPAC) issued guidelines for transmission-based precautions in hospitals. In addition to precautions for BBP, airborne, droplet and contact isolation procedures were also included. Under this regime, procedures to protect health services personnel from BBP are referred to as Standard Precautions, previously identified as Universal Precautions. All CG Health Services will adopt the use of standard blood and body fluid precautions as recommended by the CDC and OSHA.

2. Policy.

   a. Health services personnel. Health services personnel will adhere to infection-control principles, general hygiene measures, and the Center for Disease Control and Prevention's (CDC's) "standard precautions" to prevent transmitting infectious disease between themselves and their patients.

   b. Mandatory vaccination. Hepatitis B vaccination is mandatory for all CG active duty and reserve members and all civilian health care providers. The civilian administrative staff is exempt; however, these personnel are encouraged to receive Hepatitis B vaccination. Civilian clinic administrative personnel declining to receive Hepatitis B vaccination must sign this statement on an Chronological Record of Care, Form SF-600, and it shall be retained in the individual's health record:

   > I understand due to my occupational exposure to blood or other potentially infectious materials I may be at risk of acquiring Hepatitis B virus (HBV) infection. I have been given the opportunity to be vaccinated with the Hepatitis B vaccine, at no charge to myself. However, I decline Hepatitis B vaccination at this time. I understand that by declining this vaccine, I continue to be at risk of acquiring hepatitis B, a serious disease. If, in the future, I continue to have occupational exposure to blood or other potentially infectious materials and I want to be vaccinated with Hepatitis B vaccine, I can receive the vaccination series at no charge to me.

   c. Emergency Medical Technicians. Emergency Medical Technicians will adhere to the "standard precautions" described in Chapter 13-J-3.

   d. OSHA Blood-Borne Pathogen (BBP) Standard. Under the OSHA Blood-Borne Pathogen (BBP) Standard, all health services administrative and clinical personnel are potentially occupationally exposed. All clinics shall provide the health care professional responsible for vaccinating employees with Hepatitis B vaccine a copy of the OSHA BBP Standard.

3. Standard Precautions.

   a. Background. Since medical history and examination cannot reliably identify all patients infected with HIV or other blood-borne pathogens, health services personnel must consistently use blood and body-fluid precautions with all patients, including those in emergency care settings in which the risk of blood exposure is greater and the patient's infectious status usually is unknown. CDC currently recommends the "standard blood and body-fluid precautions" approach or "standard precautions."

   (1) All health care workers will routinely use appropriate barrier precautions to prevent skin and mucous membrane exposure when anticipating contact with any patient's blood or other body fluids. Personnel will wear gloves to touch patients' blood and body fluids, mucous membranes, or broken skin; to handle items or surfaces soiled with blood or body fluids; and to perform venipuncture and other vascular access procedures. Personnel

will change gloves after contact with each patient. Personnel will wear masks and protective eyewear or face shields during procedures likely to generate blood droplets or other body fluids to prevent exposure to oral, nasal, or optic mucous membranes. Personnel will wear gowns or aprons otherwise identified under Personal Protective Equipment (PPE) during procedures likely to generate blood splashes or other body fluids. All protective clothing must be removed before leaving the work area.

(2) Hand Hygiene

  (a) During the delivery of healthcare, avoid unnecessary touching of surfaces in close proximity to the patient to prevent both contamination of clean hands from environmental surfaces and transmission of pathogens from contaminated hands to surfaces.

  (b) When hands are visibly dirty, contaminated with proteinaceous material, or visibly soiled with blood or body fluids, wash hands with either a nonantimicrobial soap and water or an antimicrobial soap and water.

  (c) If hands are not visibly soiled, or after removing visible material with nonantimicrobial soap and water, decontaminate hands in the clinical situations described in Paragraph 2-c-(1-6). The preferred method of hand decontamination is with an alcohol-based hand rub. Alternatively, hands may be washed with an antimicrobial soap and water. Frequent use of alcohol-based hand rub immediately following handwashing with nonantimicrobial soap may increase the frequency of dermatitis. Perform hand hygiene:

    (1) Before having direct contact with patients.

    (2) After contact with blood, body fluids or excretions, mucous membranes, nonintact skin, or wound dressings.

    (3) After contact with a patient's intact skin (e.g., when taking a pulse or blood pressure or lifting a patient).

    (4) If hands will be moving from a contaminated-body site to a clean-body site during patient care.

    (5) After contact with inanimate objects (including medical equipment) in the immediate vicinity of the patient.

    (6) After removing gloves.

(3) All health services personnel will take precautions to prevent injuries caused by needles, scalpels, and other sharp instruments or devices during procedures or when cleaning used instruments, disposing of used needles, and handling sharp instruments after procedures. To prevent needle stick injuries, personnel will not by hand directly recap needles, purposely bend or break them, remove them from disposable syringes, or otherwise manipulate them. After using disposable syringes and needles, scalpel blades, and other sharp items, personnel will dispose of them by placing

them in puncture-resistant containers located as close to the use area as practical. The CG prohibits the use of reusable needles.

(4) Per CFR 1910.1030 Subpart Z (2001), OSHA requires: a) the use of sharps protection devices with engineered sharps injury protection, b) evaluation by employers with input from non-managerial employees involved in the use of the devices, and c) documentation of efforts to implement requirements. Employers must consider, and where appropriate, use effective engineering controls. Effective being defined as a device, that based on reasonable judgment, will make an exposure incident less likely to occur in the application in which it is used. The evaluation and documentation shall include the following:

(a) Methods of evaluation.

(b) Results of evaluation.

(c) Justification for selection decision.

(5) Although research has not definitively implicated saliva in HIV transmission, it is prudent to use appropriate protective barriers such as mouthpieces, resuscitation bags, or other ventilation devices instead of direct mouth-to-mouth resuscitation. These devices must be available for use in areas where the need for resuscitation is predictable.

(6) Health care workers who have exuding lesions or weeping dermatitis will not provide any direct patient care or handle patient care equipment until the condition resolves.

(7) Eating, drinking, smoking, applying cosmetics or lip balm, and handling contact lenses are prohibited in work areas with a reasonable likelihood of occupational exposure to BBP.

(8) Personnel shall not keep food and drink in refrigerators, freezers, shelves, drug storage areas, or cabinets or on counter tops or bench tops where blood or other potentially infectious materials are present.

(9) Personnel shall perform all procedures involving blood or other potentially infectious materials in a manner that prevents droplets of these substances from splashing, spraying, and splattering.

(10) Pregnant health care workers apparently do not face greater risk of contracting HIV infection than non-pregnant health care workers; however, if a health care worker develops HIV infection during pregnancy, the infant risks infection due to prenatal or perinatal transmission. Therefore, pregnant health care workers will thoroughly learn and strictly adhere to standard precautions to minimize the risk of HIV transmission.

b. Implementation. Implementing standard blood and body fluid precautions for all patients eliminates the need for the "Blood and Body Fluid Precautions" isolation category CDC previously recommended for patients known or suspected to be infected with blood-borne pathogens. Personnel will use isolation precautions as necessary if they diagnose or suspect associated conditions, such as infectious diarrhea or tuberculosis.

4. Precautions for Invasive Procedures.

   a. Aseptic techniques. Acceptable aseptic techniques are to be used by all persons in the surgical area. Environmental controls are implemented to ensure a safe and sanitary environment.

   b. When to use standard precautions. The standard blood and body fluid precautions listed above and those listed below shall be the minimum precautions for all invasive procedures, defined as surgical entry into tissues, cavities, or organs; repair of major traumatic injuries in an operating or delivery room, emergency department, or out-patient setting, including both physicians' and dentists' offices; a vaginal delivery; manipulating, cutting, or removing any oral or perioral tissues, including tooth structure, during which bleeding occurs or the potential for bleeding exists.

   c. Types of precautions. All health care workers who routinely participate in invasive procedures shall take appropriate barrier precautions to prevent skin and mucous membrane contact with all patients' blood and other body fluids. Personnel shall wear gloves and surgical masks for procedures that commonly generate droplets, splash blood or other body fluids, or generate bone chips, such as those using rotary dental instrumentation. Personnel shall wear gowns or aprons made of materials that provide an effective barrier during invasive procedures likely to splash blood or other body fluids.

   d. Accidents. If a glove is torn, cut, or punctured, the wearer will remove it, re-scrub, and put on a new glove as promptly as patient safety permits. The needle or instrument involved in the incident shall also be removed from the sterile field.

5. Precautions for Medical Laboratories. Blood and other body fluids from all patients will be considered infectious. To supplement the standard precautions listed above; the following precautions are recommended for health care workers in clinical laboratories.

   a. Blood and body fluid specimens. All blood and body fluid specimens shall be placed in a well-constructed, labeled container with a secure lid to prevent leaking during transport, taking care when collecting each specimen to avoid contaminating the container's exterior or the laboratory form accompanying the specimen.

   b. Equipment. All persons obtaining or processing blood and body fluid specimens (e.g., removing tops from vacuum tubes) shall wear gloves. Personnel shall wear masks and protective eyewear if they anticipate contact with mucous membrane with blood or body fluids, change gloves, and wash hands after completing specimen processing.

   c. Routine procedures. For routine procedures such as histological and pathologic studies or microbiologic culturing, a biological safety cabinet is not necessary. However, personnel shall use biological safety cabinets (Class I or

II) whenever performing procedures with a high potential for generating droplets, including activities such as blending, sonicating, and vigorous mixing.

d. Pipetting. Use mechanical pipetting devices to manipulate all liquids in the laboratory. Never pipette by mouth.

e. Needles. When using needles and syringes, personnel will follow the recommended standard precautions to prevent needle injuries.

f. Decontamination. Decontaminate laboratory work surfaces with an appropriate chemical germicide after spilling blood or other body fluids and completing work activities. Decontaminate contaminated materials used in laboratory tests before reprocessing or place such materials in bags and dispose of them according to institutional policies for disposing of infectious waste. Decontaminate scientific equipment contaminated with blood or other body fluids with an appropriate chemical germicide and clean such equipment before repairing it in the laboratory or transporting it to the manufacturer.

g. Hand washing. All persons shall wash their hands after completing laboratory activities and remove protective clothing before leaving the laboratory.

6. Handling Biopsy Specimens. Generally, personnel must put each specimen in a sturdy container with a secure lid to prevent leaking during transport and take care when collecting specimens to avoid contaminating the container's exterior. If the outside of the container is visibly contaminated, clean and disinfect it or place it in an impermeable bag before delivery to the appropriate destination for examination.

7. Using and Caring for Sharp Instruments and Needles.

a. Sharps. Personnel will consider sharp items (needles, scalpel blades, dental burs, and other sharp instruments) potentially infectious and handle them with extreme care to prevent unintentional injuries.

b. Disposal items. All generating personnel must place disposable syringes, tube holders, needles, scalpel blades, anesthetic carpules and other sharp items in closable, leak-proof, puncture-resistant containers. Cardboard containers are not appropriate for this purpose. To prevent unintentional needle stick injuries, personnel will not directly recap disposable needles by hand, purposefully bend or break needles, remove them from disposable syringes or tube holders, or otherwise manipulate them after use.

(1) At the discretion of the Health Services Administrator, a clinic may elect to receive sharps from patients for proper disposal. If so, then the following criteria must be met.

(a) The sharps container must be:

[1] Installed in a non-sensitive area to allow for disposal by patients.

[2] Accessible by wheelchair bound patients.

[3] Out of the reach of children.

[4] Maintained regularly and replaced when ¾ full.

    (b) Patients must dispose of their own sharps into an appropriate sharps container.

    (c) Patients will be instructed to maintain lancets, needles, and other sharps in a leak-proof, puncture-resistant container such as a bleach container or 2-liter soda bottle.

  (2) The Health Services Administrator must maintain policies and procedures for the handling of sharps brought into the clinic.

c. Recapping needles. If multiple injections of anesthetic or other medications from a single syringe are required, personnel may use these techniques in lieu of directly recapping by hand:

  (1) Use an approved shielding device specifically designed to recap safely (e.g., "On-Guard").

  (2) Use the "scoop" recapping technique. Affix the empty needle sheath to a flat surface and "scoop" it onto the exposed needle. A hand does not touch the sheath until the needle is securely inside.

  (3) Use a hemostat to recap by securing the empty sheath well away from the health care worker's hand.

d. Needle sticks protocol. All CG Health Care Units shall establish a needle stick protocol; see Chapter 13-J-14. If a needle stick occurs, the affected person shall report the accident to his or her immediate supervisor, who will document the incident in a memorandum to the SHSO or health services department head, with a copy to the affected person. The memorandum will detail the needle stick's time, date, and circumstances and any medical treatment received. The SHSO or health services department head shall ensure the established needle stick protocol is observed in all cases.

8. Infection Control Procedures for Minor Surgery Areas and Dental Operatories.

a. Medical History. Always obtain a thorough medical history. For dental procedures, have the patient complete a Dental Health Questionnaire, Form CG-5605. Amplify this information by asking the patient specific questions about medications, current illnesses, hepatitis, recurrent illness, unintentional weight loss, lymphadenopathy, oral soft tissue lesions, results of last HIV test, or other infections. Completely review the individual's health record or consult with a physician if the history reveals active infection or systemic disease.

b. Using Personal Protective Equipment and Barrier Techniques.

  (1) Health services personnel (HCW) in CG medical/dental treatment facilities must comply fully with 29 CFR, Part 1910, OSHA Occupational Exposure to Blood Borne Pathogens. OSHA has determined that health care workers face a significant health risk as a result of occupational exposure to blood and "other potentially infectious materials" (OPIM) that

may contain potentially harmful blood borne pathogens. This risk can be minimized or eliminated by the practice of standard precautions including the use of PPE.

(2) PPE is defined in CFR 1910.1030 as specialized clothing worn by an employee for protection against a blood borne hazard. PPE must be removed daily, when visibly soiled, or when leaving the work area and must be commercially laundered at the unit's expense. Under no circumstances shall employees take PPE or contaminated clinic attire from the workplace for self-laundering.

(3) Health services personnel will consider all patients' blood, saliva, and other body fluids infectious. To protect themselves and patients, personnel must always wear gloves when touching:

(a) Blood.

(b) Saliva.

(c) Body fluids or secretions.

(d) Items or surfaces contaminated by the above.

(e) Mucous membranes.

(4) Further, personnel must completely treat one patient, if possible, and wash and re-glove hands before performing procedures on another patient. Repeatedly using a single pair of gloves is not allowed; such use can produce defects in the glove material, which reduce its effectiveness as a barrier to microorganisms. Additionally, when gloves are torn, cut, or punctured, the wearer immediately must remove them, thoroughly wash his or her hands, and put on new gloves before completing minor surgical or dental procedures.

(5) Personnel shall wear surgical masks and protective eyewear or a chin-length plastic face shield. Personnel shall change masks after lengthy examinations or procedures, most especially after any, which produce spatter. Patient protective eyewear shall be provided during all treatment procedures likely to splash or spatter blood, saliva, gingival fluids, or foreign objects. Personnel will use rubber dams, pre-procedural mouth rinsing, high-speed evacuation, and proper patient positioning, when appropriate, to minimize droplet generation and spatter in the dental operatory.

(6) Clinic attire is defined in Paragraph 10.

c. Hand Hygiene.

(1) Hand hygiene includes hand washing, alcohol-based hand rubs, and surgical/aseptic hand washing. Wearing gloves does not replace the need for hand hygiene.

(2) Indications for hand hygiene are: before and after treating patients (e.g. before glove placement and after glove removal), after barehanded

touching of inanimate objects likely to be contaminated by blood or saliva, before regloving after removing gloves that are torn, cut, or punctured, and before leaving the dental operatory.

(3) At the beginning of the day, hand washing with plain soap is adequate, since soap and water will remove transient microorganisms. Wet hands with water, apply product, rub hands together for at least 15 seconds, rinse and dry with a disposable towel. Whenever possible wash hands at sinks that provide hot and cold water through a single mixing valve.

(4) During the rest of the day, for routine dental procedures, alcohol-based hand rubs are recommended. Apply product to palm of one hand, rub hands together covering all surfaces until dry. The appropriate volume of product is based on manufacturer. Alcohol based hand rubs should NOT be used if hands are visibly soiled or contaminated.

(5) For surgical procedures, personnel must use an antimicrobial surgical hand scrub. Scrub hands and forearms for the length of time recommended by manufacturer (2-6 minutes). Clinics may need to stock non-allergenic soap and sterile gloves for allergic individuals.

(6) Health services personnel who have exuding lesions or weeping dermatitis must refrain from all direct patient care and handling patient-care equipment until the condition resolves.

(7) Health services personnel should avoid wearing artificial nails and keep natural nails short as to minimize harboring bacterial growth.

d. Dental equipment. Sterilizing and Disinfecting Dental Hand Pieces, Ultrasonic Scalers, Dental Units, and Dental Laboratory equipment by the following procedures:

(1) After each use with each patient, personnel will sterilize dental hand pieces (including high-speed, low-speed components used intra-orally and ultrasonic scalers) because the device may aspirate a patient's blood, saliva, or gingival fluid into the hand piece or waterline. Clinics should purchase sufficient numbers of autoclavable hand pieces to meet this requirement. Dry heat is the recommended method of sterilizing dental burs.

(2) Disinfect all dental unit surfaces with a suitable chemical germicide between patients or cover such surfaces during use. Use impervious backed paper, aluminum foil, or clear plastic wrap to cover surfaces difficult or impossible to disinfect (e.g., light handles or x-ray tube heads). Remove the covering while gloved, discard the covering, remove used and don fresh gloves, and then recover with clean material after each patient.

(3) Dental laboratory personnel will observe infection control protocols. They will thoroughly, carefully clean blood and saliva from material used in the mouth (e.g., impression materials, occlusal registrations), especially before polishing and grinding intra-oral devices. They will clean and disinfect contaminated materials, impressions, and intra-oral devices before

COMDTINST M6000.1F

handling them in the dental laboratory and before putting them in a patient's mouth. They will disinfect laboratory instruments (e.g. spatulas, knives, and wax carvers), plastic benches, chucks, handles, switches, tubing, air hoses, and lab hand pieces every day. Rubber mixing bowls require overnight immersion to disinfect. Workstations, including exposed equipment, drawers, work surfaces, and sinks, require weekly surface disinfecting. Because of the increasing variety of dental materials used intra-orally, dental providers should consult with manufacturers about specific materials' stability in disinfecting procedures.

e. Dental Unit Waterlines.

(1) Background: Studies have demonstrated that dental unit waterlines are colonized with a wide variety of microorganisms including bacteria, fungi, and protozoa. Microorganisms colonize and multiply on the interior surfaces of the waterlines resulting in the formation of biofilms. Although oral flora may enter and colonize dental water systems, the public water system is the primary source of the microorganisms found in waterline biofilms.

(2) Discussion: Current dental water systems cannot deliver water of optimal microbiologic quality without some form of intervention by the user. The literature supports the need for improvement in dental unit water quality. Improving the microbiologic quality of water used in dental treatment shows commitment to high-quality patient care. All CG dental clinics should take prudent measures to provide quality water for dental treatment and to ensure a safe and healthy environment for their patients and employees.

(3) All CG dental clinics shall follow the Centers for Disease Control and Prevention (CDC) recommendation that only sterile solutions be used for surgical procedures that involve the cutting of bone.

(4) The number of colony forming units (CFU) in water used as a coolant or irrigant for non-surgical dental treatment should be as low as reasonably achievable. The ceiling limit for acceptable dental water quality is ≤ 500 CFU/mL of heterotrophic plate count bacteria, the regulatory standard for safe drinking water. Non-surgical procedures include most subgingival scaling or restorative procedures and for initial access into the dental pulp.

(5) Water Quality Improvement: There are several options for improving dental unit water quality. They are:

(a) Flushing: Flush waterlines for 2-3 minutes at the beginning of the day, 20-30 seconds between patients to eliminate any retracted oral fluids, and 3 minutes at the end of the day. Mechanical flushing is an interim measure and has no effect on biofilms. However, flushing between patients will remove patient material potentially retracted during treatment, and should be continued even when other methods to control biofilms are used.

(b) All water lines should be completely drained and air purged at the end of the day. This procedure will remove all existing water, dry the lines and discourage the re-growth of microorganisms.

(c) An independent water reservoir will eliminate the inflow of municipal water into the dental unit and provides better control over the quality of source water for patient care. Independent water reservoirs are available as optional equipment on most new dental units and can be retrofitted to existing equipment. Use of independent reservoirs when used with a routine disinfection protocol, can virtually eliminate bacterial and fungal contamination.

(d) Periodic monitoring should be performed to assess compliance with recommended protocols and to identify technique errors or non compliance. Dental staff should be trained regarding water quality, biofilm formation, water treatment methods, and appropriate maintenance protocols for water delivery systems. Clinical monitoring of water quality can ensure that procedures are correctly performed and that devices are working in accordance with the manufacturer's previously validated protocol. Dentists should consult with the manufacturer of their dental unit or water delivery system to determine the best method for maintaining acceptable water quality (i.e., $<$/= 500 CFU/mL) and the recommended frequency of monitoring.

(e) If the dental unit manufacturer does not provide a recommendation for frequency of monitoring then monthly testing on a semi-random basis is recommended, (e.g. daily, weekly, monthly so it is easy to remember to perform the testing). Water should be tested at each exit point of the unit. If a unit fails to test $<$/=500 CFU/mL, the unit shall be re-treated (under supervision if need be). This does not preclude the continued use of the dental unit.

(f) Monitoring of dental water quality can be performed by using commercial self-contained test kits or commercial water-testing laboratories. Because methods used to treat dental water systems target the entire biofilm, no rationale exists for routine testing for such specific organisms as *Legionella* or *Pseudomonas*, except when investigating a suspected waterborne disease outbreak.

f. Dental Radiology Sterilization and Disinfecting Procedures.

(1) Sensor-Holding and Aiming Devices. Sensor-holding and aiming devices will be heat-sterilized.

(2) Panoramic Unit Bite Blocks. Use disposable bite block covers between patients. If disposable covers are not available, treat bite blocks similarly to sensor-holding devices.

(3) Digital radiography sensors and other high-technology instruments (e.g., intraoral camera, electronic periodontal probe, occlusal analyzers, and lasers) come into contact with mucous membranes and are considered

semicritical devices. They should be cleaned and ideally heat-sterilized or high-level disinfected between patients. However, these items vary by manufacturer or type of device in their ability to be sterilized or high-level disinfected. Semicritical items that cannot be reprocessed by heat sterilization or high-level disinfection should, at a minimum, be barrier protected by using an FDA-cleared barrier to reduce gross contamination during use. To minimize the potential for device-associated infections, after removing the barrier, the device should be cleaned and disinfected with an EPA-registered hospital disinfectant (intermediate-level) after each patient. Manufacturers should be consulted regarding appropriate barrier and disinfection/sterilization procedures for digital radiography sensors, other high-technology intraoral devices, and computer components.

(4) X-ray Chair. Between patients wipe arm- and headrests with a chemical surface disinfecting solution. If using paper or plastic headrest covers, replace them after each patient.

(5) Intra-oral X-ray Tubehead and Exposure Buttons. Wipe these items with a surface disinfectant or cover them after each patient visit. Do not allow disinfectant liquid to leak into the tubehead seams or the exposure button switch.

(6) Digital Sensors. Digital sensors will be covered with a disposable plastic sleeve.

9. Sterilizing and Disinfecting.

   a. Background. The rationale for sterilization is to kill all microbes remaining on the instruments and help assure patient safety.

   b. Instrument Categories (Spaulding Classification). The Spaulding Classification defines as critical instruments that normally penetrate soft tissue, teeth, or bone (e.g., forceps, scalpels, bone chisels, scalers, surgical burs, etc.). They must be heat-sterilized after each use. Instruments not intended to penetrate soft or hard tissues (e.g., amalgam carvers, plastic instruments, etc.) but which may come into contact with tissues are semi-critical and also should be heat-sterilized after each use. If heat sterilization is not possible, semi-critical instruments must receive chemical sterilization. Non-critical instruments never contact tissue. Sterilization is recommended for non-critical instruments, but high-level disinfection is acceptable.

   c. Instrument Processing.

      (1) Designate a central processing area and divide into:

         (a) Receiving, cleaning, and decontamination.

         (b) Preparation and packaging.

         (c) Sterilization.

         (d) Storage.

(2) <u>Cleansing Instruments</u>. Instruments must be cleansed for sterilization to be effective. Use automated cleaning equipment (ultrasonic cleaner, instrument washer). Use a container or wrapping material compatible with then type of sterilization process. <u>Hand-scrubbing instruments is prohibited</u>. Persons who cleanse instruments must wear heavy-duty ("Nitrile") rubber utility gloves to reduce the risk of injury. Inspect instruments for cleanliness before preparing them for packaging. Use only FDA-cleared medical devices for sterilization.

(3) <u>Packaging and Wrapping Instruments</u>. Depending on intended use, wrap or package most instruments individually or in sets. Packaging in metal or plastic trays reduces set-up time; instruments and other materials arranged systematically are more convenient. Package size and sterilization method generally determine the best wrapping material, most commonly paper/plastic peel pouches, nylon plastic tubing, cloth, sterilization wrap, or wrapped cassettes. Seal packages by heat, tape, and self-sealing methods. Wrap instruments loosely to allow the sterilizing agent to circulate freely throughout the pack. Pack scissors, hemostats, and hinged instruments in the open position so the sterilizing agent can reach all parts. When wrapping in an easily punctured material, cover the tips of sharp instruments with 2 x 2 gauze or cotton roll. If using plastic or nylon sterilization tubing, the pack should be approximately 20% larger than the longest instrument to allow the inside air to expand when heated. Clear tubing is relatively puncture-resistant and enables rapid identification of contents. When using cloth to wrap critical items, use a double thickness. Package instruments/cassettes with microbial barriers. Allow packages to dry in the sterilizer before they are handled to avoid contamination. Do not use liquid chemical sterilants for surface disinfection or as holding solutions.

d. <u>Heat Sterilization</u>. The best way to minimize cross-contamination is to sterilize all instruments that can withstand sterilizing conditions. The most practical, dependable sterilization method, heat, when appropriate, is preferable to chemical means. These are the most common heat sterilization techniques:

(1) <u>Steam Vapor under Pressure Sterilizer (Autoclave)</u>. Steam vapor under pressure is an excellent sterilization method. Moist heat kills the bacteria by causing their proteins to denature and coagulate within the microbial cell. The steam's high temperature, not the pressure, kills the microorganisms. Steam can rust cutting edges made of carbon steel; however, antirust agents reduce this process.

(2) <u>Chemical Vapor under Pressure Sterilizer (Chemiclave)</u>. This sterilizer uses chemical vapor under pressure and kills bacteria in much the same manner as the steam sterilizer. It is an excellent sterilization method. Because chemical vapors are less corrosive than steam, they do not dull sharpened instruments. Chemical vapor sterilizers use a specific mixture of formaldehyde, alcohols, ketone, acetone, and water. If the

manufacturer's recommended chemical solution is not available, distilled water may be used for a short time. Chemical solutions shall be used only once. A disadvantage of the chemical vapor sterilizer is the residual chemical vapor that escapes into the air when the chamber door is opened. While non-toxic and non-mutagenic, its odor can be objectionable. Allowing the sterilizer to cool for at least 20 minutes before opening will significantly reduce the residual vapor level. A commercial purging system that reduces residual vapor levels is available.

(3) <u>Dry Heat Sterilizer</u>. Dry heat kills bacteria by an oxidation process. Dry heat sterilization will not corrode instruments, but dry heat sterilizers can destroy metal instruments' temper and melt solder joints if not monitored properly. Some dry heat units are not able to sterilize large trays and require special wrapping and bagging materials. For these reasons, dry heat sterilization is not recommended for critical instruments, and should be monitored carefully and used judiciously with semi-critical and non-critical instruments. Because sterility is destroyed as soon as items are touched or left open to the environment, do not place loose instruments in dry heat sterilizers. Wrap and bag all instruments; they must remain wrapped or bagged until used.

e. <u>Sterilization Monitoring</u>.

(1) All sterilization procedures must be monitored and recorded in a log book for compliance.

(2) <u>Mechanical Monitoring</u>. Correct time, temperature and pressure is monitored to demonstrate that the physical parameters of the sterilization process have been achieved with every load. Use mechanical monitoring with each load.

(3) <u>Chemical Monitoring</u>. Chemical indicators show that every package has been exposed to sterilizing conditions in a heat sterilizer. They do not guarantee the instruments are sterile. External chemical indicators (autoclave tape or sterilizing bags with heat-sensitive printing) identify at a glance which instruments have been processed but show that only the outside of the pack was exposed to an elevated temperature. An external chemical indicator must be on every pack processed. If using see-through packages, a chemical indicator placed inside the pouch is acceptable. Internal chemical indicators, available in strips, cards, or labels, react to time/temperature/ sterilizing agent combinations – use an internal chemical indicator inside each package. Do not use instrument packages if mechanical or chemical indicators suggest inadequate processing.

(4) <u>Biological Monitoring (Spore testing)</u>. Bacterial spores are used to demonstrate that the sterilization procedure kills highly resistant microbes (bacterial spores). Place them in the most challenging area of the load being tested and wrap the pack in the usual fashion. Monitor all chemical vapor, water vapor, and dry heat sterilizers with a spore test either weekly or each cycle, whichever is less frequent.

(a) These systems require either a medical laboratory service or an in-house incubator to incubate the test spore. Dry heat sterilizers require an alternate system using a glassine envelope with enclosed spore strips. Regardless of the system used, document spore monitoring, including identification test date, test results, and operator, and maintain the records for two years.

(b) In the case of a positive spore test, take the sterilizer out of service and review procedures to determine if operator error could be responsible. Re-test the sterilizer using biological, chemical, and mechanical indicators after correcting any procedural problems. If repeat test is negative and the chemical and mechanical tests are normal, put the sterilizer back in service. If the repeat spore test is positive do not use the sterilizer until it has been inspected or repaired or the problem identified. Recall and reprocess items from the suspect loads. Re-test the sterilizer with spore tests in three consecutive empty chamber sterilization cycles after the cause of the failure has been determined and corrected before putting it back into service.

(5) Storage and Shelf Life. Implement practices based on date- or event-related shelf life for the storage of wrapped, sterilized items. Materials are considered indefinitely sterile unless packaging is torn, ripped, punctured or exposed to water. At a minimum, place the date of sterilization and which sterilizer was used on the package. Examine wrapped sterilized packages before opening them to ensure the barrier wrap is intact. Re-clean, re-pack and re-sterilize packages that are compromised. Store sterile packages in dry closed cabinets.

f. Chemical Sterilization and High-Level Disinfection.

(1) Although heat is the preferred sterilization method, certain instruments and plastics will not tolerate heat sterilization and require chemical sterilization or high-level disinfection. These disinfectants destroy microorganisms by damaging their proteins and nucleic acids. Most formulae contain 2% glutaraldehyde and come in two containers. Mixing the proper amounts from each container activates the solution. Sterilization monitors cannot verify glutaraldehyde sterilization. The solution is caustic to the skin, so use forceps or rubber gloves to handle instruments immersed in glutaraldehyde and *always* follow manufacturer's directions *carefully*. Label each container of fresh solution with an expiration date.

(2) Uninterrupted immersion for 7 to 10 hours in a fresh glutaraldehyde solution usually will achieve sterilization; uninterrupted immersion for 10 minutes will kill most pathogenic organisms, but not spores. Heavily soiled or contaminated instruments render glutaraldehydes ineffective. Debride instruments thoroughly to disinfect effectively. Glutaraldehydes are not recommended for surface disinfection.

g. Surface Disinfection.

(1) Extraordinary efforts to disinfect or sterilize environmental surfaces such as walls, floors, and ceilings generally are not required because these surfaces generally do not transmit infections to patients or health care workers. However, routinely clean and remove soil from them.

(2) After contamination, wipe all other treatment room surfaces such as countertops, dental chairs, light units, exam tables, and non-sterile objects in the operating field with absorbent toweling to remove any extraneous organic material, and then disinfect them with a suitable chemical germicide. Personnel shall wear heavy-duty ("Nitrile") rubber utility gloves when applying surface disinfectants. Many different chemical disinfectants possessing varying degrees of effectiveness are available. The following three surface disinfectants are recommended.

(a) Iodophor. Iodophor compounds contain 0.05 to 1.6% iodine and surface-active agents, usually detergents, which carry and release free iodine. Iodophor's antimicrobial activity is greater than that of iodine alone: 10 to 30 minutes of contact produces intermediate levels of disinfection. Iodophors are EPA-approved as effective when diluted 1:213 with water. Because iodine's vapor pressure is reduced in iodophor, its odor is not as offensive. In addition, iodophors do not stain as readily as iodine.

(b) Phenolics. In high concentrations, phenolic compounds are protoplasmic poisons. In low concentrations, they deactivate essential enzyme systems. As disinfectants, phenolics are usually combined with a detergent; 10 to 20 minutes of contact produces disinfection. Phenolics are less corrosive to treated surfaces.

(c) Sodium Hypochlorite. Sodium hypochlorite is thought to oxidize microbial enzymes and cell wall components. A 1:10 dilution of 5.25% sodium hypochlorite in water produces a solution which disinfects at an intermediate level in 10 minutes. Sodium hypochlorite solution tends to be unstable, so prepare a fresh solution daily. It possesses a strong odor and can harm eyes, skin, clothing, upholstery, and metals (especially aluminum).

(3) Chemical Disinfectants Not Recommended For Use.

(a) Alcohol. Alcohol is bactericidal against bacterial vegetative forms by denaturing cellular proteins. Diluted in water, a 70 to 90% solution is more effective than a more concentrated solution. Alcohol's disadvantages are: (1) rapid evaporation, (2) lack of sporicidal or viricidal activity, and (3) rapid inactivation by organic material. Since alcohol interferes with proper surface cleansing, it has no place in the disinfection protocol.

(b) Quaternary Ammonium Compounds. In the past, benzalkonium chlorides and other "quats" were used as disinfectants because they were thought to be safe and inexpensive and have low surface tension. Their biocidal activity breaks down the bacterial cell membrane, producing an altered cellular permeability. As a group, these compounds have serious deficiencies. Being positively charged, they are attracted to not only bacteria but also to glass, cotton, and proteins, which decrease their biocidal activity. Common cleaners, soaps, and other compounds negatively charged ions neutralize "quats." Research has shown some "quats" support the growth of gram-negative organisms. Quats are ineffective against most spore formers, the Hepatitis B virus, and the tubercle bacillus.

10. <u>Clinic Attire</u>.

a. <u>Definition</u>. Clothing ensembles worn during routine direct patient encounters when not anticipating exposure to blood or OPIM is considered clinic attire.

b. <u>Approved clinic attire</u>. Approved clinic attire is defined as military uniforms or surgical scrubs only. Clinical attire is NOT intended to be PPE and must be supplemented by PPE whenever exposure to blood or OPIM is reasonably anticipated. Surgical scrubs worn as clinic attire shall be worn in designated direct patient care work areas of the clinic, only when engaged in direct patient care activities and shall not be worn outside the clinic. Undergarments worn under scrubs will be the same as those required to be worn under military uniforms. Under no circumstances should long-sleeve undergarments be worn. When arms need to be covered when performing procedures, long sleeve PPE should be worn. The work area is defined in OSHA BBP plan as the area where potential blood borne exposure exists, including corridors or passageways in direct patient care areas.

c. <u>Soiled Clinic attire</u>. Clinic attire that is visibly soiled with blood, OPIM or that had been exposed to contaminated spray or splatter is considered contaminated. PPE is always considered contaminated even if no visible evidence of contamination is present. At no time shall PPE or contaminated clinic attire be worn in administrative areas, break areas, or areas where food or potable drink are stored, prepared or consumed.

d. <u>PPE or contaminated clinic attire</u>. Except for commercial laundering, PPE or contaminated clinic attire shall not be removed from the clinic's direct patient care area, nor shall it be stored in personal clothing lockers nor removed from the clinic.

e. <u>Name tags</u>. When wearing surgical scrubs, military uniforms and civilian clothing as clinical attire, HCWs must also wear a name tag that includes name, rank and occupation (i.e. Physician, Dentist, Physician Assistant, Nurse Practitioner, and Health Service Technician) clearly visible to all patients.

11. <u>Storage and Laundering of Clinic Attire, PPE and Linen</u>.

a. <u>Laundering clinic attire and PPE</u>. Military uniforms and civilian clothing worn as clinic attire that is visibly soiled with blood or OPIM or have been exposed to contaminating spray and spatter is considered contaminated laundry and shall be commercially laundered only at the expense of the unit. PPE is considered contaminated even if no visibly evidence of contamination is present and shall be commercially laundered at the expense of the unit. All linen shall be commercially laundered at the expense of the unit. All surgical scrubs, even if not contaminated will not be taken home for self-laundering and shall be commercially laundered only at the expense of the unit.

b. Handling contaminated laundry. Contaminated laundry, including scrubs, shall be placed and transported in bags labeled or color-coded in accordance with OSHA Regulation, Bloodborne Pathogens Standards, 1910.1030(g)(1)(i). (If contaminated laundry is wet, bags or containers must prevent leakage or soak-through). Gloves and other appropriate PPE will be worn when handling contaminated laundry.

c. Linen. Although research has identified soiled linens as a source of large numbers of certain pathogenic microorganisms, the risk of linens actually transmitting disease is negligible. When handling soiled linen, it is recommended to always wear gloves. Handle it as little as possible and with minimum agitation to prevent gross microbial contamination of the air and persons handling the linen. Carefully check linen for sharps objects and remove them before washing. Bag all soiled linen where used; do not sort or rinse it in patient care areas.

12. Cleaning and Decontaminating Blood or Other Body Fluid Spills. Use an EPA-approved germicide or recommended surface disinfectant agent to promptly clean all blood and blood-contaminated fluid spills. Health care workers must wear gloves. First remove visible material with disposable towels or other appropriate means that prevent direct contact with blood. If anticipating splashing, wear protective eyewear and an impervious gown or apron that provides an effective barrier to splashes. Next decontaminate the area with disinfectant solution or an appropriate EPA-approved germicide. Clean and decontaminate soiled cleaning equipment or put it in an appropriate container and dispose of it according to clinic policy. Use plastic bags clearly labeled as containing infectious waste to remove contaminated items from the spill site. Remove gloves; then wash hands.

13. Infectious Waste.

a. Medical waste. Epidemiological evidence does not suggest most clinic waste is any more infectious than residential waste. However, public concern about the risk of medical wastes must not be ignored. Identifying wastes for which special precautions are necessary include those wastes which potentially cause infection during handling and disposal and for which special precautions appear prudent, including sharps, microbiology laboratory waste, pathology waste, and blood specimens or products. While any item that has touched blood, exudates, or secretions potentially may be infectious, it is usually not considered practical or necessary to treat all such waste as infectious. Materials containing small amounts of blood, saliva, or other secretions such as tainted gauze pads, sanitary napkins, or facial tissues are not considered infectious waste. Generally, autoclave or incinerate infectious waste before disposing of it in a sanitary landfill. Infectious waste autoclaving standards are different from normal sterilization standards. Carefully pour bulk blood, suctioned fluids, excretions, and secretions down a drain connected to a sanitary sewer. Or for materials capable of it, grind and flush such items into sanitary sewers (some states prohibit this practice).

b. Environmental Protection Agency classification. The Environmental Protection Agency classifies health care facilities as generators of infectious waste based on the weight of waste generated. CG classification is based on facility type. All CG clinics are considered generators. Each CG health care facility must have a written infectious waste management protocol consistent with state and local regulations in the unit's area.

c. Biohazard. Biohazard warning labels shall be affixed to regulated waste containers; refrigerators, and freezers containing blood or other potentially infectious material; and other containers used to store, transport, or ship blood or other potentially infectious materials with these exceptions:

(1) Substitute red bags for labels on regulated waste bags or containers. OSHA believes red bags protect personnel because they must comply with OSHA BBP Standard Paragraph (g)(2)(iv)(M), which requires training personnel to understand the meaning of all color-coding.

(2) Individual containers of blood or other potentially infectious materials placed in a labeled container during storage, transport, shipment or disposal.

14. Managing Exposures (Bloodborne Pathogen Exposure Control).

a. Exposure.

(1) An exposure occurs if a health care worker comes in contact with blood or other body fluids in one of these ways:

(a) Parenteral—through a needle stick or cut;

(b) Mucous membrane—from a splash to the eye or mouth;

(c) Cutaneous—contact with large amounts of blood or prolonged contact with blood when the health care worker's exposed skin is chapped, abraded, or afflicted with dermatitis.

(2) After an exposure, if the source of the exposure is known, obtain the source person's consent (if applicable), making sure to follow local laws governing consent for testing non-active duty source persons and incompetent or unconscious persons.

(3) The treating healthcare provider will perform an initial screening of the exposure incident to determine if the "source" is known to be HIV positive. This should be done within 15 minutes of the exposure. If the "source" is known to be HIV positive, the treating physician will contact the nearest hospital with infectious disease services, notify them of the exposure and arrange a time for the exposed worker to be seen ASAP.

(4) Post-exposure prophylaxis (PEP) should be initiated as soon as possible, preferably within hours rather than days of exposure. If a question exists concerning which antiretroviral drugs to use, or whether to use a basic or expanded regimen, the basic regimen should be started immediately rather than delay PEP administration. The optimal duration of PEP is unknown, however the CDC recommends a 4 week period for PEP. The nearest local hospital with infectious disease services should be consulted for additional guidance.

(5) If the HIV status of the source is not known, a rapid HIV antibody test should be performed on the source at the nearest local hospital or USMTF (protocol for clinic use of rapid HIV antibody testing will be developed soon). Each clinic should have a local hospital point of contact who can assist with obtaining stat HIV results. Viromed should not be utilized for stat testing because the results will not be available until 48 hours post-exposure. If the test is positive, the treating physician should prescribe HIV PEP based on CDC guidelines.

(6) In addition to determining the HIV status of the source, a blood sample should be drawn and tested for, Hepatitis B Surface Antigen, Hepatitis C Antibody, and for the ALT status of the source person. Provide the source person post-test counseling and treatment referrals. Inform the exposed person of the source person's test results and applicable laws and regulations on disclosing the source person's identity and infectious status. It is extremely important all persons who seek consultation for any HIV-related concerns receive appropriate counseling from a USMTF or other medical facility capable of providing this service.

(7) After an exposure, any worker (active duty, civilian, or contractor) incurring an exposure to blood/body fluids will wash or flush the area for at least 5 minutes, and then report the exposure immediately to their supervisor. The exposed individual is to then to seek medical attention immediately. Workers reporting to an outside facility initially should follow-up at a CG clinic on the next day (during regular business hours).

(8) Recommendations for Hepatitis B PEP and HIV PEP are located in Paragraph 14-b and c. Currently, there is no recommendation for Hepatitis C PEP. Both active duty and civilian workers will be followed by the local CG clinic. Contract workers will be contacted by a healthcare provider to educate them on their need to follow-up with their private physician and to provide them the results on the "source".

(9) All clinics shall ensure the health care professional evaluating a worker after an exposure incident has this information:

(a) A copy of the OSHA BBP Standard;

(b) A description of the exposed employee's duties as they relate to the exposure incident;

(c) Documentation of the route(s) of exposure and circumstances under which exposure occurred; and

(d) Results of the source individual's blood tests, if available; and all records on the employee's appropriate treatment, including vaccination.

(10) The SME shall obtain and give the exposed person a copy of the evaluating health care professional's written opinion within 15 days after the evaluation is complete. The healthcare professional's written opinion for post-exposure evaluation and follow-up shall be limited to the following:

(a) Written opinion for Hepatitis B vaccination shall be limited to whether Hepatitis B vaccination is indicated for an employee, and if the employee has received such vaccination.

(b) The employee has been informed of the results of the evaluation.

(c) The employee has been told about any medical conditions resulting from exposure to blood or other potentially infectious materials which require further evaluation or treatment.

(11) A copy of the SME's written opinion will also be provided to the SHSO or health services department head. The QI coordinator or his or her designee also will retain a copy and ensure all required follow-up treatment and testing is documented. The SHSO or health services department head shall ensure that the following this management protocol is adhered.

(12) Utilize Bloodborne Pathogen Exposure Guidelines, Form CG-6201.

b. <u>Hepatitis B Virus Post-exposure Management</u>.

(1) For a worker exposed to a source individual found to be positive for HbsAg:

(a) The exposed worker who has not previously received Hepatitis B vaccine will receive the vaccine series. A single dose of Hepatitis B immune globulin (HBIG) if it can be given within 7 days of exposure is also recommended.

(b) Test the exposed worker who has previously received Hepatitis B vaccine for antibody to Hepatitis B surface antigen (anti-HBs). If the antibody level in the worker's blood sample is inadequate (i.e., less than 10 SRU by RIA, negative by EIA) give the exposed employee one dose of vaccine and one dose of HBIG.

(2) If the source individual is negative for HbsAg and the worker has not been vaccinated, the worker shall receive Hepatitis B vaccination.

(3) If the source individual refuses testing or cannot be identified, the unvaccinated worker should receive the Hepatitis B vaccine series. Consider administering HBIG on an individual basis if the source

individual is known or suspected to be at high risk of HBV infection. At his or her discretion the responsible Medical Officer will manage and treat as needed previously vaccinated workers who are exposed to a source who refuses testing or is not identifiable.

 (4) Additional guidance on Hepatitis B PEP be found at the CDC Updated USPHS Guidelines for the Management of Occupational Exposures to HBV, HCV, and HIV and Recommendations for Postexposure Prophylaxis, MMWR, June 29, 2001 / 50(RR11):1-42 – http://www.cdc.gov/mmwr/preview/mmwrhtml/rr5011a1.htm

 c. Human Immunodeficiency Virus Post-exposure Management.

  (1) Workers who have an occupational exposure to HIV should receive follow-up counseling, post-exposure testing, and medical evaluation regardless of whether they receive PEP. In view of the evolving nature of HIV post-exposure management, the health care provider should refer to Coast Guard Human Immunodeficiency Virus (HIV) program, COMDTINST M6230.9 (series).

15. Training Personnel for Occupational Exposure. All Health Services Divisions or Branches will inform and train personnel in occupational exposure initially on assignment and annually thereafter. Personnel who have taken appropriate training within the past year need to receive additional training only on subjects not previously covered. The training program shall contain at least these elements:

 a. An accessible copy and explanation of the regulatory text of this standard (Federal Register 56 (235): 64175, December 6, 1991 [29 USC 1910.1030]).

 b. A general explanation of the epidemiology and symptoms of bloodborne diseases.

 c. An explanation of bloodborne pathogen transmission modes.

 d. An explanation of the exposure control plan outlined in Chapter 13-J.

 e. An explanation of the appropriate methods to recognize tasks and other activities that may involve exposure to blood and other potentially infectious materials.

 f. An explanation of methods to reduce or prevent exposure, such as barrier techniques, and their limitations.

 g. Information on the types and properly using, locating, removing, handling, decontaminating, and disposing of personal protective equipment.

 h. An explanation of the basis for selecting personal protective equipment.

 i. Hepatitis B vaccine. Information on the Hepatitis B vaccine, including efficacy, safety, administration, and benefits. This vaccination is mandatory for active duty and reserve personnel.

j. Information on appropriate actions to take and persons to contact in an emergency involving blood or other potentially infectious materials.

k. Explanation of the procedures. An explanation of the procedure to follow if an exposure incident occurs, including the method of reporting the incident and available medical follow-up described in Chapter 13-J-13.

l. Information on the post-exposure evaluation and follow-up the Senior Medical Officer (SMO) or designee is required to provide for the employee after an exposure incident.

m. An explanation of the signs, labels, and/or color coding required for sharps and biohazardous materials.

n. A question-and-answer period with the person conducting the training session.

K. <u>Patient Safety and Risk Management Program</u>.

1. <u>Purpose</u>.

   a. <u>Background</u>. The patient safety and risk management program supports quality medical care by identifying, analyzing, and preventing actual and potential risks to patients and staff. The program provides mechanisms to detect and prevent medical errors, accidents and injuries and reduces the cost of claims and loss of other resources. Patient safety involves a variety of clinical and administrative activities that identify, evaluate and reduce the potential for harm to beneficiaries and to improve the quality of health care.

   b. <u>Responsibilities</u>. Patient safety and risk management programs are most effective if they are prospective, preventive, and comprehensive. All staff members, beneficiaries, contract providers, and volunteers shall be aware of risks in the clinical environment and act safely and responsibly to implement program requirements. Patient safety and risk management activities are not limited to claims activities but examine all instances of actual and potential risk or loss. Successful patient safety programs facilitate a non-punitive, interdisciplinary approach to decrease unanticipated adverse health care outcomes. The organizational focus is on continued learning about risks and risk management strategies and reengineering systems/processes to reduce the chance of human error.

2. <u>Informed Consent</u>.

   a. <u>Background</u>. Every person, with a few exceptions, has the right to be examined and treated only in the manner they authorize. This individual prerogative is based on the concept a competent patient has the right to make informed decisions about health care. Consent for health care must be informed, voluntary, competent, and specific, and is clearly an important issue in quality patient care. The objective of informed consent is improved patient-provider communication in non-emergent situations, which should result in patients' realistic expectations about the nature of treatment and the expected outcome, and reduced liability for the government. Clear documentation demonstrating the patient was properly informed is necessary to protect the patient, the provider, and the government. Although patients must be informed of treatment options, military members who refuse treatment necessary to render them fit for duty (including immunization) are subject to separation and/or disciplinary action (see Chapter 2-A-4.-b.).

   b. <u>Responsibilities</u>.

      (1) SHSO: The SHSO must publish facility-specific implementing instructions that ensure providers carry out the spirit and intent of this Section. The SHSO and HSWL SC should monitor compliance with consent policies and procedures as a regular part of medical and dental records review.

  (2) Health Care Providers: Responsible health care providers must counsel patients before treatment and document receiving the patient's informed consent.

 c. <u>Types of Consent</u>.

  (1) Expressed Consent: This type of consent is obtained by open discussion between the provider and patient and must include a statement the patient consents to the proposed procedure. Expressed consent may be oral or written.

  (2) Oral Consent. Except where this regulation specifically requires written consent, oral consent is sufficient authorization for treatment. However, oral consent is difficult to prove. If a health care provider receives oral consent to treatment, he or she must document it by an entry in the treatment record. Consent received from competent authority by telephone is a form of oral expressed consent; a person not directly involved in the patient's care should witness such consent; and it must be documented by an entry in the treatment record.

  (3) Conditions Requiring Written Consent. Document written consent by having the patient sign forms authorizing treatment and including an entry in the treatment record that discusses the requirements outlined in Chapter 13-K-4. Except in emergencies, written consent is required for these situations:

   (a) All surgical procedures (including, among others, placing sutures, incision and drainage, removing a foreign body(s), cauterizing, removing wart(s), injecting medications into a joint(s), etc.)

   (b) Invasive tests and procedures to diagnose and treat disease or remove tissue specimens (e.g., biopsies), except routine phlebotomy.

   (c) Anesthesia, including local dental anesthesia.

   (d) All dental procedures.

   (e) Genitourinary procedures including vasectomies, IUD insertion or removal, etc.

 d. <u>Implied Consent</u>. Implied consent is derived from the patient's conduct even if he or she does not communicate specific words of consent. Assume implied consent only if one can reasonably presume the patient knows the risks, benefits, and alternatives to treatment. For example, a patient's presence at dental sick call is implied consent for a dental exam. Never accept implied consent to treatment involving surgical therapy or invasive diagnostic procedures except in emergencies.

e. Emergencies. Consent before treatment is not necessary when immediate. treatment is required to preserve the patient's life or limb. The provider will document the existence and scope of the emergency and describe the events precluding obtaining consent.

f. Who May Consent. Generally, competent adult patients who have the capacity to manage their own affairs who present themselves for treatment have the authority to consent. If a patient is incompetent due either to statutory incompetence (e.g., a minor) or mental impairment, then it must determined who the individual with legal capacity to consent and obtain his or her consent before examining or treating the patient. Laws defining minors and to what they may legally consent differ by state. The law of the state where the facility is located governs legal capacity to consent. Each clinic will develop a policy for treating minors.

g. Information to Provide. The provider must advise the patient of the nature of his or her condition; describe the proposed treatment in terms the patient can understand; and explain the material risks and expected benefits of the proposed treatment course, available alternative health care options, and the option of non-treatment. A material risk is one a reasonable person likely would consider significant in deciding whether to undertake therapy and is a function of the likelihood of occurrence, the severity of the injury it threatens to cause, and existing reasonable alternatives. A provider is not required to explain risk that are considered extremely remote unless the patient requests an explanation or the potential adverse consequences are so grave a reasonable person in the patient's particular circumstances would consider the risk important.

h. Informing the Patient. Health care providers will provide information in a manner that allows a patient of ordinary understanding to intelligently weigh the risks and benefits when faced with the choice of selecting among the alternatives or refusing treatment altogether. Health care providers must communicate in language one can reasonably expect the patient to understand. Although open discussions between the responsible health care provider and the patient should be the standard, each department may develop internal methods to acquaint patients with the benefits, risks, and alternatives to procedures requiring consent. In some departments, prepared pamphlets or information sheets may be desirable.

i. Documentation. Regardless of the method used to inform the patient or the form of consent (oral or written), the provider must document the disclosure and the patient's reactions in the medical or dental record. It is highly recommended to document this in progress notes even if the patient has signed a preprinted "consent" form. Progress notes written to document disclosing information to the patient will be specific about the information provided. The notes must specifically enumerate risks, alternative forms of treatment, and expected benefits the provider discussed with the patient. Use the

Request for Administration of Anesthesia and for Performance of Operations and Other Procedures, Form SF-522 to document consent in all surgical, anesthetic and reproductive procedures.

j. Witness to Consent. All consent forms require a witness's signature. The witness may be a health care facility member who is not participating in the procedure or treatment. Patients' relatives are not acceptable as witnesses. The witness confirms the patient signed the form, not that he or she received all relevant information.

k. Duration of Consent. Consent is valid as long as no material change in circumstances occurs between the date the patient consented and the procedure or treatment date. Obtain new consent if a material change in circumstances occurs, for example the provisional diagnosis changes. If more than seven (7) days elapse between the date the patient signed the consent and the date treatment begins, provider and patient must re-sign, re-initial, and re-date the consent form. A new consent is not required for each stage in a series of treatments for a specific medical condition (e.g., repeated application of liquid nitrogen to warts).

3. Adverse Event Monitoring and Reporting.

   a. Definitions.

      (1) Action Plan: The end product of a Root Cause Analysis that identifies the risk reduction strategies to prevent the recurrence of similar adverse events.

      (2) Adverse Event: An occurrence or condition associated with the provision of health care or services that may result in harm or permanent effect. Adverse events may be due to acts of omission or commission. Incidents such as falls or erroneous administration of medications are also considered adverse events even if there is no harm or permanent effect.

      (3) Contributing Factors: Additional reasons for an event or series of events that may result in harm, which could apply to individuals, systems operations or the organization.

      (4) Near Miss: An event or situation that could have resulted in harm but did not either by chance or timely intervention.

      (5) Root Cause: The most basic reason that a situation or treatment did not turn out as planned or as expected.

      (6) Root Cause Analysis: A process for identifying the basic or contributing causal factor(s) associated with a sentinel event, an adverse event or close call. The review is interdisciplinary and includes those who are closest to the process, and focuses on systems and processes, not individual

performance. An ad hoc Root Cause Analysis Team, with membership as necessary depending on the event, is identified by the patient safety official to develop the Root Cause Analysis and Action Plan.

(7) Safety Assessment Code: A risk assessment tool that considers the severity of an adverse or near miss event together with the probability of the event's recurrence. The score, or Safety Assessment Code, assigned to the event determines the type of action that should be taken, e.g., Root Cause Analysis (score 3), intense analysis (score 2 or 1) or no action. Severity is divided into four categories – catastrophic, major, moderate, and minor. Probability is divided into three categories – high, medium, and low. This provides a standardized process for prioritizing actions and applying resources where there is the greatest opportunity to improve safety.

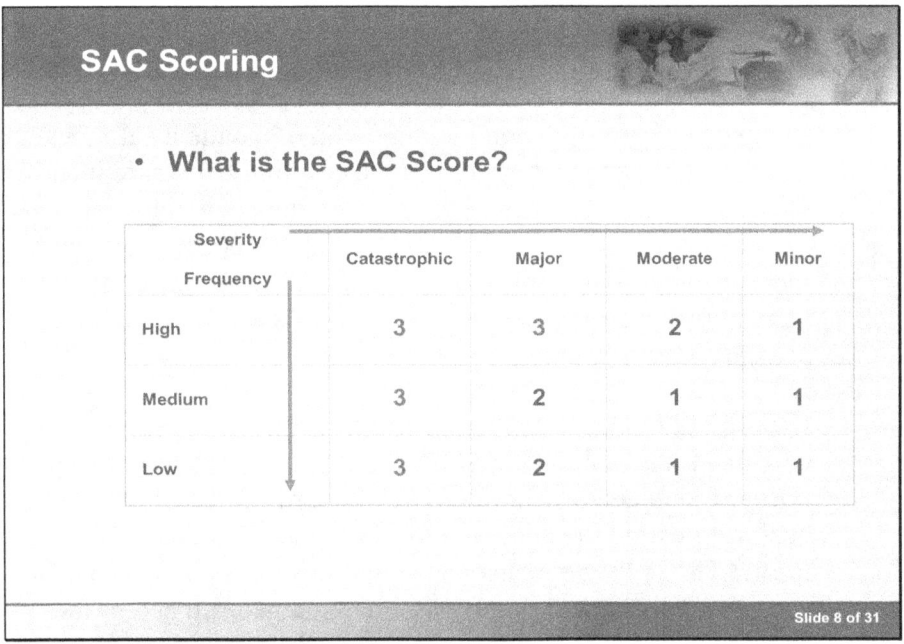

SAC Scoring

• **What is the SAC Score?**

Severity Frequency	Catastrophic	Major	Moderate	Minor
High	3	3	2	1
Medium	3	2	1	1
Low	3	2	1	1

Slide 8 of 31

Table 13-K-1

(8) Sentinel Event: An unexpected occurrence involving death or serious physical or psychological injury, or the risk thereof that is not related to the natural course of an individual's illnesses or underlying condition. Such events signal the need for immediate investigation and proactive response on the part of the organization.

b. Significant Events. Events are not reviewed to place blame or discipline those involved, but rather to assess the health care process(es) and systems involved and identify potential areas for improvements in patient safety. The CG Health Care Program uses the resulting recommendations to determine health care policy, personnel, equipment and training needs to prevent future adverse health care outcomes or patient injuries. A significant event may result in initiating a Mishap Board as the Safety and Environmental Health Manual, COMDTINST M5100.47 (series), requires and a legal investigation conducted concurrently with a medical incident review of the same event (e.g., a vessel collision with injuries). In most cases however, an adverse event review will occur solely within a CG health care facility or the CG Health Care Program.

c. Responsibilities.

    (1) SHSO: The SHSO must publish facility-specific implementing instructions that ensure providers carry out the spirit and intent of this Section.

    (2) Health Care Providers: Identification and reporting of near misses and adverse events must be encouraged as an expectation of everyday practice by CG health care. Prevention of harm to patients and reporting all potential and/or adverse events is a performance expectation for all CG health care program staff.

d. Immediate Actions. Upon identification of a patient safety event, the staff member will immediately perform necessary health care interventions to protect and support the patient(s). Practitioners will be contacted as soon as possible to report the incident and provide an update. The staff member/practitioner will take all necessary health care interventions to contain risk and to present event-related materials that may be needed for analysis or investigation.

e. Reporting Procedure. Within 24 hours after an adverse event occurs, the command shall submit copy(s) of Emergency Care and Treatment Report, Form SF-558 and/or Chronological Record of Care, Form SF-600 for events occurring within the clinic and/or Emergency Medical Treatment Report, Form CG-5214 for events occurring outside the clinic to the HSWL SC. Clearly mark "Patient Safety Report" in large print across the top of these forms. Stamp or print this statement on the top of each document: "This is a medical quality assurance document. It is protected by Federal law." HSWL SC shall send copies of the documents to Commandant (CG-112) within three days of receipt.

f. Review Procedure. On receiving one of the three forms, HSWL SC conferring with Commandant (CG-112), shall review the document(s); verify the event meets the Chapter 13-K-3 criteria for an adverse event or near miss; determine whether an on-site medical review or Root Cause Analysis shall be conducted; and designate a single point of contact at Commandant (CG-112). A Root Cause Analysis must be conducted and an Action Plan completed for all adverse events with Severity Assessment Code 3.

(1) If HSWL SC, after conferring with Commandant (CG-112), determines a medical incident review is unnecessary, they shall notify the command by letter within 10 working days of the event and send a copy of the letter to Commandant (CG-112).

(2) If an on-site medical incident review or Root Cause Analysis is indicated, HSWL SC shall notify the involved command as soon as possible and designate a clinic professional staff member to conduct a review or convene a panel of qualified professional staff members from the involved facility, to review all aspects of the incident. To ensure confidentiality, the panel shall consist of only the designated facility point of contact and the persons HSWL SC appoint.

(3) If a patient safety event is an intentional unsafe act that results from gross negligence or possible criminal activity, the event shall be reported to the appropriate authorities for investigation.

g. Incident review officer or Root Cause Analysis Team. The incident review officer or Root Cause Analysis Team shall request and review all relevant documents and reports, interview personnel as required, and when the review is complete, submit a written letter report with this information on the incident to Commandant (CG-112) through the HSWL SC:

(1) Synopsis. A brief summary of the incident and injuries and/or fatalities involved.

(2) Factual Information. Factual information and data about the incident and personnel involved shall consist of at least these topics:

(a) History. The chronological order of any significant event preceding, during, and after the incident, including any written logs or transcripts of radio logs substantiating this chronology, such as the Emergency Care and Treatment, Form SF-558, the Emergency Medical Treatment Report, Form CG-5214, or the Chronological Record of Care, Form SF-600.

(b) Injuries. Describe each injury, or in the case of fatalities, the cause of death. Include autopsy findings when available.

(c) Professional qualifications of all persons who delivered health care, if relevant, including all recent applicable training and certificates (e.g., ACLS, BLS, EMT, HS, etc.).

(d) Equipment Performance. List all pertinent medical equipment used during the incident and any failures due to mechanical malfunction, operator error, inadequate training, or other factors. Describe whether equipment involved was maintained or serviced according to manufacturers' specifications.

(e) Applicable Medical and/or Dental Guidelines.

(3) Analysis and Conclusions. The analysis and conclusion should contain the individual's or panel's hypothesis of the circumstances surrounding the event, emphasizing the health care aspect, including a brief conclusion about the health care rendered and how it contributed to the event's outcome.

(4) Action Plan. The action plan comprises recommended modifications and risk reduction strategies in policy, staffing, equipment, training, or other health care delivery system aspects that need improvement to avoid similar incidents in the future. The action plan should address responsibility for implementation, oversight, pilot testing (if appropriate), timelines and the metrics to be used in evaluating the effectiveness of the actions taken.

h. Routing Patient Safety Review Reports.

(1) The completed root cause analysis report will be sent from the clinic to Commandant (CG-112) thru HSWL SC for review and appropriate action.

(2) Staff members who submit patient safety event reports shall receive timely feedback on the actions being taken as a result of their report. Management efforts and activities shall focus on improving the systems and processes that may have contributed to the patient safety event.

(3) In cases involving an unanticipated outcome of care, a qualified health care provider shall inform the patient. QI-protected information shall not be released or provided to the patient. During the communication, at least one other health care program staff member should be present. The provider shall document in the patient's record what was communicated.

4. Patient Safety Training.

a. All health care program staff shall receive patient safety, risk management and teamwork education during their initial orientation and on an as-needed basis.

b. Patient safety topics shall include an overview of the patient safety and risk management program, roles and responsibilities in reporting patient safety events, patient education in safety and effective communication strategies.

L. Training and Professional Development.

1. Definitions.

   a. ACLS (Advanced Cardiac Life Support). Sponsored by the American Heart Association (AHA) and American Safety and Health Institute (ASHI), this 16-hour program (8 hours for recertification) emphasizes cardiac-related diagnostic and therapeutic techniques and grants a completion certificate valid for two years on completion. An ACLS certificate of completion recognizes that a person completed the course and does not in any way authorize him or her to perform skills taught there. ACLS also sometimes refers to the cardiac component of Advanced Life Support. Online ACLS courses without hands-on skills proficiency testing are not accepted substitutes for the ACLS courses noted above.

   b. Advanced Life Support (ALS). A general term applied to pre-hospital skills beyond the basic life support level including, among others, EKG interpretation, medication administration, and advanced airway techniques.

   c. Basic Life Support (BLS) for the Health Care Provider. Health care providers must successfully complete and maintain proficiency in a program sponsored by any of the following: The Military Training Network, American Heart Association (AHA), American Red Cross (ARC), American Safety & Health Institute (ASHI) or the American College of Emergency Physicians (ACEP). (The Military Training Network is the preferred choice). Successful completion grants certification for 2 years. The course curriculum of all programs includes basic skills (e.g. airway maintenance, cardiac compression and use of the automatic external defibrillator) necessary to sustain heart and brain function until advanced skills can be administered.

   d. Emergency Medical Technician (EMT). A general term referring to the certification of pre-hospital care providers. Four skill levels (EMR, EMT, EMT-Advanced, EMT-Paramedic) are recognized, but functions performed at each level vary significantly by jurisdiction. The term EMT applies to all CG personnel with EMT training and certification, regardless of rating.

   e. Paramedic. An individual certified by the National Registry of Emergency Medical Technicians as an Emergency Medical Technician-Paramedic (NREMTP) or certified by a local governing body to perform ALS procedures under a physician's license.

2. Unit Health Services Training Plan (In-Service Training).

   a. Health Services Units. These personnel must have an on-going in-service training program aimed at all providers with emphasis on the Health Services Technicians' professional development. It is expected of clinic staff members attending outside training to share new information with other staff members.

In-service training sessions allow clinics to ensure issues of clinical significance are presented to their staff.

b. Clinic Training Program must include these topics, among others.

(1) Quality Improvement Implementation Guide Exercises.

(2) Annual review of clinic protocols on suicide, sexual assault, and family violence.

(3) Patient satisfaction issues.

(4) Patient sensitivity.

(5) Patient confidentiality to include HIPAA guidelines.

(6) Emergency I.V. therapy.

(7) Emergency airway management.

(8) Cardiac monitor and defibrillator familiarization.

(9) Cervical spine immobilization and patient transport equipment.

(10) Emergency vehicle operator's training (where operated).

(11) Section 13-J: Infection and Exposure Control Program.

c. Health Services Training Coordinator (HSTC). The SHSO must designate in writing a Health Services Training Coordinator (HSTC) who coordinates clinic in-service training, distributes a quarterly training schedule, and maintains the unit's health services training record. The HSTC's responsibilities include these:

(1) Establishes and maintains a Health Services Training Record to document all training conducted within the clinic. Records should include presentation outline, title, program date, name of presenter, and list of attendees. Maintain training records for 3 years from the date on which training occurred.

(2) Ensures all emergency medical training is documented in the individual's CG Training Record, CG-5285 for credit toward the 48-hour National Registry EMT continuing education requirement.

(3) Maintains a Training Record section that records personnel certifications including CPR, ACLS, EMT, and flight qualifications, including expiration dates and copies of the current certificate. The HSTC should ensure assigned personnel obtain recertification before current certificates expire.

3. Emergency Medical Training Requirements.

   a. BLS Certification. All active duty, civilian, and contract civilian personnel working in CG clinics and sick bays shall maintain current BLS certification at the health care provider level (AHA "C" Course or equivalent).

   b. SAR or MEDEVAC. Every Health Services Technician who participates in SAR or MEDEVAC operations must be a currently certified EMT by NREMT. The Flight Surgeon may authorize, in writing, EMTs to perform BLS and ALS skills in the course of their assigned SAR/MEDEVAC duties.

   c. Emergency Vehicles. At least one currently certified EMT will staff CG Emergency Vehicles. CG Emergency Vehicles will only be required to meet ambulance standards, as defined by Federal Specification KKK-A-1822E and as defined under CFR 42 Part 410 Section 41 when staffed by paramedics and specified as an ambulance service. For HSWL RP facilities staffed only by HSs with an EMT designation, ambulances shall not be provided/utilized and only an unmarked general purpose vehicle will be available to convey Emergency Responders to scenes outside of the clinic. Stable patients with minor injury/illness not requiring transport off-site to a hospital may be transported as a passenger back to the clinic in the general purpose vehicle. General-purpose vehicles shall not be equipped with emergency warning lights and/or sirens nor shall they display a "star of life" insignia or other emblem implying emergency medical capabilities.

   d. ACLS Certification. All Medical Officers serving in clinical assignments will maintain current ACLS certification. Only licensed or certified physicians, nurse practitioners, physician assistants, or nationally registered advanced life support providers (EMT-P and EMT-I) will perform advanced life support (ALS) procedures, except as Chapter 13-L-3-e stipulates. Paramedics may perform functions authorized by their certifying jurisdiction's protocols with written Medical Officer authorization. Other than those described this section, persons who have completed an ACLS course should note certification means only they have completed the course and does not convey a license to perform any skill. Individuals completing ACLS courses shall serve as a clinic resource on current standards for pre-hospital care in training and equipment areas. ACLS classes that are electronic only (e-ACLS) do not satisfy this certification requirement. Individuals with documented training and demonstrated proficiency may request and obtain written authorization by a local CG Medical Officer to perform emergency medical procedures not normally associated with EMT-B skill sets (e.g. use of Combitube).

   e. EMT training (basic course or recertification). HSs must possess current National Registry EMT certification in order to be eligible for advancement to E-4, E-5, E-6, or E-7. Training and continuing education sources available to meet this requirement, and certification criteria, are discussed below.

Effective 1 October 1990, the NREMT became the certification standard for all new or recertifying CG EMS Providers.

(1) Forward requests for training (EMT initial or EMT recertification) via the chain of command to the local unit's Training Officer for submission of the member's Electronic Training Request (ETR) to be entered into Direct Access (DA). Commandant (CG-1121), using the ETR, will identify and select individuals for training based upon the unit requirements, quota availability, number of qualified EMT personnel already assigned, and member's rotation/expiration of enlistment dates. Nonrated members will not routinely be selected due to possible early rotation for Class "A" schools. Members striking a rating for a unit billet, however, will be considered. Once the TONO is issued, unit commanding officers must request authority to substitute personnel from Commandant (CG-1121) via email, with information copy to Training Quota Center.

(2) If pursuing local training sources, programs must meet the Department of Transportation (DOT) National Standard Curriculum guidelines and offer National Registry certification. Units will fund, or request District funding for travel costs associated with the use of local Basic or recertification EMT courses. Tuition costs associated with these courses, if any, will be funded by Commandant (CG-1121) for designated personnel. For local training courses with tuition costs, proceed as per paragraph 13.L.3.e.(1).

4. Health Services Technician "A" School.

a. FORCECOM operates the introductory course for Health Services Technicians, including the Emergency Medical Technician (EMT) course, at TRACEN Petaluma. As program manager, Commandant (CG-1121) provides professional inputs to the TRACEN on curriculum and qualifying requirements. FORCECOM manages HS "A" School personnel quotas. The Training and Education Manual, COMDTINST M1500.1(series), outlines selection requirements and procedures.

b. All HS "A" School students must successfully pass the NREMT examination in order to advance to HS3 upon graduation.

5. Health Services Technician "C" Schools.

a. Training. Due to the specialized nature of health care, the CG requires some Health Services Technicians to complete training in medical specialty fields such as aviation medicine, preventive medicine, medical and dental equipment repair, physical therapy, laboratory, radiology, pharmacy, and independent-duty specialties. The usual sources are Department of Defense training programs and through IDHS training which is conducted at CG Training Center Petaluma.

b. Selection for HS "C" Schools. Selection for HS "C" Schools is based on qualification code requirements for HS billets at clinics and independent duty sites as specified in personnel allowance lists. Secondary selection criteria include command requests, personnel requests, and deficiencies noted on HSWL SC Quality Improvement Site Surveys.

   c. Training Request. Applications for Class "C" School training shall be submitted via Electronic Training Request (ETR) in Direct Access by the Unit Training Officer or as specified by the program. The member and Unit Training Officer are responsible for ensuring all pre-requisites are met and the member's current position requires the training. If a unit submits an ETR, it is expected that prerequisites are met and the unit is confident that the trainee will be available for training on the dates requested. HS personnel wishing to pursue "C" school training in courses of 20 weeks or longer require a permanent change of duty station coordinated by Commander, Personnel Service Center (PSC-epm-2).

6. Continuing Education Programs.

   a. Licensing. All PHS and CG Physician Assistants must maintain active professional licenses and/or certification to practice their professional specialty while assigned to the CG. Licensing and/or recertification requirements often demand continuing professional education, which enhances the practitioner's skills and professional credentials.

   b. Funding. The Director of Health and Safety encourages one continuing education course annually for all licensed health services professionals. The funding command using HSC 30 funds will approve the Short Term Training Requests. This program is in addition to the operational medicine (AFC 56) training program (see Chapter 1 of this Manual). Generally training should provide at least six documented continuing education credits per day pertinent to the applicant's CG billet. Personnel should obtain training at the nearest possible geographic location.

   c. Licensing and Certification Exams. Medical and Dental Officers' licensing and certification exams will not be funded as continuing education. CG-sponsored Physician Assistant (PA) programs' graduates may request funding for examination fees (primary care only), travel to the testing site nearest their current duty station, and per diem associated with obtaining initial certification from the National Commission on Certification of Physician Assistants. The CG funds this one-time exception because it sponsors the PA training program and requires certification for employment. PA's may take the recertification examination in conjunction with the annual physician assistant conference. Travel and per diem will be authorized as annual CME. The member pays recertification examination fees.

   d. Healthcare Provider Training. There are several required medical, dental, leadership, CBRNE, and Disaster training courses. These are listed at http://www.uscg.mil/hq/cg1/cg112/cg1121/medtraining.asp.

e. Procedures. Except for Health Service Technician "C" School applicants, Health and Safety Program personnel requesting continuing education must follow these procedures:

(1) Applications for training shall be submitted via Electronic Training Request (ETR) in Direct Access by the Unit Training Officer or as specified by the program. The member and Unit Training Officer are responsible for ensuring all pre-requisites are met and the member's current position requires the training. If a unit submits an ETR, it is expected that prerequisites are met and the unit is confident that the trainee will be available for training on the dates requested.

(2) Accompany each training request with course literature (e.g., a descriptive brochure) or a brief written description.

(3) Submit Request, Authorization, Agreement and Certification of Training, Form SF-182 (10 parts) with proper endorsements if using a government purchase order to pay tuition or fees.

(4) Send all completed forms to Commandant (CG-112) for processing.

(5) Training requests must arrive at Commandant (CG-112) 8 weeks before the anticipated training convening date. Coast Guard Training Quota Management Center (TQC), Portsmouth, VA, processes approved requests and issues orders.

7. Long-Term Training Programs.

a. Long-Term Post-Graduate Training. Long-Term Post-Graduate Training for Medical Officers (Physicians, Physician Assistants, and Nurse Practitioners). This 1- to 2-year program for Medical Officers principally emphasizes primary care (family practice, general internal medicine). Consideration may be given for non-primary care specialties such as sports medicine, occupational health, public health, and preventive medicine. Training in orthopedics is a potential option for mid-level practitioners only. The Health Services Program Manager will consider non-primary care post-graduate medical training only when needed. Applicants also must have applied to their chosen training program and meet its requirements before requesting training. Applicants should have served with the CG Health Services Program for at least 2 years for each year of training received. For physician applicants, highest consideration will be given first to those who have not completed an initial medical residency. Commandant (CG-112) has more information.

b. Comprehensive Dental Residency. This 2-year program provides Dental Officers advanced training in general dentistry, enabling them to give more effective, comprehensive dental care to CG beneficiaries. The Naval Postgraduate Dental School, National Naval Medical Center, Bethesda, MD, conducts the training, designed to qualify Dental Officers to meet the American Dental Association and the American Board of General Dentistry requirements for specialty board examination. Dental Officers chosen for this program are expected to pursue board certification. For program prerequisites and applications procedures, see the Training and Education Manual, COMDTINST M1500.1 (series).

c. Health Services Administration. This program provides instruction in facility and personnel management, program planning, cost containment, quality assurance, third-party payment and liability, and medical-legal issues. The program provides training at the undergraduate (bachelor's degree) level for Chief Warrant Officers and senior enlisted HS personnel (Medical Administrators) and post-graduate (master's degree) level for officers in grades O-2, O-3, and O-4. See the Training and Education Manual, COMDTINST M1500.1 (series) for eligibility requirements, prerequisites, and application procedures.

d. Physician Assistant Program. Conducted at the U.S. Inter-service Physician Assistant Program, Fort Sam Houston TX, this program trains CG personnel interested in becoming Physician Assistants. Program graduates receive a baccalaureate degree from the University of Nebraska. If they meet eligibility requirements, graduates are offered a direct commission as ensigns as described in the Officer Accessions, Evaluations, and Advancements, COMDTINST M1000.3 (series). Each year, up to three Coast Guard students are selected for training based on Service needs. Training at other institutions is not authorized. See the Training and Education Manual, COMDTINST M1500.1 (series) for eligibility requirements, prerequisites, and application procedures.

M. Patient Affairs Program.

1. Patient Sensitivity.

   a. The importance of patient sensitivity. The CG considers patient sensitivity issues of paramount importance in delivering health care. Important issues in this area include medical record confidentiality, appropriate privacy during medical examination and treatment, respect for patient concerns and cultural backgrounds, and enhancing the patient's perception of the quality of services delivered. Patients are always treated with respect, consideration and dignity.

   b. Training. All clinics shall conduct continuing patient sensitivity training.

2. Patient Advisory Committee (PAC).

   a. Purpose of the PAC. The CG's health services program provides primary health care to a wide array of beneficiaries authorized by law and regulation. Medical Treatment Facilities (MTFs) often are unaware of their population's health problems until patients voice complaints or criticisms to the command. To enable beneficiaries to express their concerns, a PAC must be available to open lines of communication between health care providers and care recipients.

   b. Each CG MTF shall establish a PAC and specify criteria for committee functions. PACs shall include one officer and one enlisted member not assigned to the clinic; an active duty representative from each CG command in the clinic's service area; an active duty representative from each of the other uniformed services using the MTF; a retired representative; and an active duty dependent representative from both officer and enlisted communities.

   c. Meeting Frequency. MTF shall conduct PAC meetings at least quarterly.

   d. The SHSO or his or her designee shall chair the meeting. Meeting minutes shall include recommended actions and an attendance list; and will be forwarded to the CO with a copy to each PAC member. Specific PAC objectives include:

      (1) Advise the SHSO on the range of services the beneficiary population requires.

      (2) Serve as a communications link between the MTF and the beneficiaries the members represent.

      (3) Serve as patient advocacy groups to assure all patients are accorded their rights as described in the Commandant's Patient Bill of Rights and Responsibilities.

      (4) Patients are provided, to the degree known, complete information concerning their diagnosis, evaluation, treatment and prognosis. When it is medically inadvisable to give such information to a patient, the information is provided to a person designated by the patient or to a legally authorized person.

(5) Patients are given the opportunity to participate in decisions involving their healthcare, except when such participation is contraindicated for medical reasons.

(6) Assist the SHSO in advising patients of their responsibilities as described in the Commandant's Patient Bill of Rights and Responsibilities. Patients are informed about procedures for expressing suggestions to the organization and policies regarding grievance procedures and appeals.

(7) Assist the SHSO in establishing patient education programs.

(8) Advise the SHSO on the acceptability and convenience of the services provided.

3. <u>Patient Satisfaction Assessment</u>.

   a. <u>Patient satisfaction</u>. Assessing patient satisfaction through patient satisfaction surveys has become an effective, efficient method to investigate and measure the quality of the CG health care delivery system from the patient's perspective.

   b. <u>Satisfaction Form Availability</u>. A patient satisfaction survey form shall be available to every patient who receives care at a CG facility. Locally prepared patient satisfaction surveys are authorized for use. Additionally, patient satisfaction surveys are randomly sent to patients from MERS. These surveys are linked to peer review for the same patient encounter and used to assess the encounter from both peer review and patient satisfaction viewpoints.

   c. <u>Survey Frequency</u>. Satisfaction surveys are randomly generated from MERS for each provider and sent to patients to complete. The frequency of surveys is variable based on number of patient visits, with goal of 100 visits per year. Patients will not be sent more than 1 survey each quarter to eliminate potential survey fatigue.

   d. <u>Patient satisfaction survey results</u>. Patient satisfaction survey results shall be provided to the quality improvement focus group for discussion and action and will be documented in meeting minutes. Survey results shall be reported and actions for improvement recommended to the unit CO, HSWL SC, and Commandant (CG-1122).

   e. <u>Care received from civilian providers</u>. Persons distant from a CG clinic can comment about care received from civilian providers by sending a mail-in HSWL SC survey form available from unit Health Services Technicians.

4. <u>Patient Grievance Protocol</u>.

   a. <u>Overview</u>. The CG expects health services personnel to maintain a professional attitude at all times. Our goal to provide the highest quality health care within allotted resources to all beneficiaries with the least personal inconvenience. Despite our best efforts, occasionally a patient will be dissatisfied with the care received.

b. <u>Individuals with grievances</u>. Whenever possible individuals with grievances should seek out or be referred to the clinic supervisor, health benefits advisor (HBA), or Health Services Administrator (HSA) for complaint resolution before leaving the clinic. Refer written or telephone complaints to the appropriate clinic staff member. At a minimum, the complainant shall be given the name of his or her unit Patient Advisory Committee representative, and the time and place of the next PAC meeting.

c. <u>Chain of command</u>. If the clinic supervisor, HBA, or CA cannot resolve the complaint, he or she shall refer the complainant to the senior medical or dental officer as appropriate.

d. <u>Unresolved complaint</u>. Refer the complainant to the CO or higher authority only if the patient believes the clinic or PAC has not resolved the complaint.

e. <u>Review of complaint</u>. HSWL SC shall review concerns reported on forms mailed to the HSWL SC for quality improvement purposes, action, or referral to an appropriate level for resolution and follow up.

5. <u>Congressional Inquiries</u>.

a. <u>Congressional liaison staff</u>. Occasionally, circumstances arise in which beneficiaries exercise their right to solicit assistance from their elected Congressional Representative to resolve their complaint with the CG health care system. The CG maintains a Congressional liaison staff to direct inquiries to the appropriate Headquarters office that can best address the issue and respond satisfactorily. Normally Commandant (CG-11) replies to health care problems.

b. <u>Investigation</u>. Congressional inquiries require a complete investigation of the circumstances surrounding the issues the beneficiary addresses. To this end, the command, health care facility, and individuals involved must supply supporting documentation and/or statements to assist in the investigation.

6. <u>Patient Bill of Rights and Responsibilities</u>.

a. <u>Posting the Bill of Rights</u>. Each CG health care facility shall conspicuously display the Commandant's "Patient Bill of Rights and Responsibilities."

b. <u>Health Services Administrator's responsibility</u>. The "Patient Bill of Rights and Responsibilities" is periodically reviewed and updated by Commandant (CG-1122). The Health Services Administrator shall assure that the most recent edition of the "Patient Bill of Rights and Responsibilities" is displayed in the clinic.

CHAPTER 14

MEDICAL INFORMATION SYSTEM (MIS) PROGRAM

CHAPTER FOURTEEN – MEDICAL INFORMATION SYSTEM (MIS) PROGRAM

A. Medical Information Systems (MIS) Plan.

1. Purpose. The Medical Information System (MIS) program described here follows the policy established by the Office of Health Services Commandant (CG-112), outlines systems and assigns responsibility for the administration of the MIS. The MIS is a key component for the overall management of CG clinics and sickbays. MIS is a dynamic tool, which will provide a comprehensive electronic solution for tracking operational medical readiness, health systems management, and patient access to care. The Health and Safety Directorate, HSWL SC, unit COs, and health care providers are responsible for ensuring successful implementation of the CG MIS.

2. Background.

   a. There is an ongoing need for Commandant, Area Commanders, and field level COs to assess medical and dental operational readiness. As one of the offshoots of this need, along with assurance of medical safety, the President and Congress have mandated the use of the Electronic Health Record (EHR) in military services. Additionally, the CG Health Services program needs to accurately capture workload, performance, and productivity through standardized methodology. Proper analysis of health care data provides the ability to realign assets where they are most needed to deliver timely, quality health care. The full implementation of the Composite Health Care System (CHCS), the military EHR, Armed Forces Health Longitudinal Technology Application (AHLTA), Medical Readiness Reporting System (MRRS), Dental Common Access System (DENCAS), and future enhancements to AHLTA will significantly enhance our ability to provide this information as needed.

   b. Federal statutes impose strict requirements for managing government information. The most pertinent Federal statutes that govern information include:

      (1) Federal Records Act (Public Law 81-754): Sets policy for and mandates establishment of agency programs for the management of Federal records.

      (2) Freedom of Information Act (Public Law 90-23): Provides policy to ensure public access to Federal government information.

      (3) Paperwork Reduction Act (Public Law 96-511): Recognizes information as a Federal resource and directs agencies to establish specific programs for management of the resource and associated elements.

      (4) Paperwork Reduction Reauthorization Act (Public Law 99-500): Defines information resources management and directs further program management requirements.

(5) A suspected or confirmed breach/compromise shall be reported in accordance with the Privacy Incident Response, Notification, and Reporting Procedures for Personally Identifiable Information (PII), COMDTINST 5260.5 (series).

(6) Privacy Act (Public Law 93-579): Provides policy and safeguards to protect privacy of individuals.

(7) Health Insurance Portability and Accountability Act (HIPAA), (Public Law 104-191): Requires health plans to assure the security and privacy of individually identifiable health information, and to use specified standards and code sets for electronic transactions involving medical information.

3. Privacy rights. CG policy concerning the privacy rights of individuals and the CG's responsibilities for compliance with operational requirements established by The Coast Guard Freedom of Information (FOIA) and Privacy Acts Manual, COMDTINST 5260.3 (series), Privacy Act and HIPAA are as follows:

a. Privacy.

(1) Protect, as required by the Privacy Act of 1974, as amended, and HIPAA, the privacy of individuals from unwarranted intrusion. Individuals covered by this protection are living citizens of the US and aliens lawfully admitted for permanent residence.

(2) Collect only the personal information about an individual that is legally authorized and necessary to support CG operations. Disclose this information only as authorized by the Privacy Act and HIPAA, and described in Chapter 4 of this Manual.

(3) Keep only personal information that is timely, accurate, complete, and relevant to the purpose for which it was collected.

(4) Safeguard personal information to prevent unauthorized use, access, disclosure, alteration, or destruction.

(5) Let individuals know what records the CG keeps on them and let them review or get copies of these records, subject to exemptions authorized by law.

(6) Permit individuals to amend records about themselves contained in CG systems of records, as authorized by HIPAA, which they can prove are factually in error, not up-to-date, not complete, or not relevant.

(7) Allow individuals to ask for an administrative review of decisions that deny them access to or the right to amend their records.

(8)   Maintain only information about an individual that is relevant and necessary for CG purposes, as required to be accomplished by statute or Executive Order.

(9) Act on all requests promptly, accurately, and fairly.

b. Security.

(1) Facility Access Controls:

(a) The CG will continually access potential risks and vulnerabilities to individual protected health information in its possession, and develop, implement and maintain appropriate administrative, physical and technical security measures in accordance with HIPAA.

(b) Clearly define the security perimeter of the premises and building. Ensure that the perimeter is physically sound. Ensure all external doors are adequately secured against unauthorized access by installing locks, alarms or other access control devices.

(c) Define the instances in which visitors are allowed, including the areas they may visit and any escort requirements.

(d) Ensure all doors to interior areas requiring compartmentalization or added security are adequately protected against unauthorized access by installing locks, alarms, or other access control devices.

(2) Workstation Use and Security

(a) Comply with all applicable CG information system security policies.

(b) Log off every time prior to leaving the terminal

(c) Inspect the last logon information for consistency with actual last logon; report any discrepancies.

(d) Comply with all applicable password policies and procedures, including not storing written passwords.

(e) Close files and systems not in immediate use.

(f) Perform memory-clearing functions to comply with security policies.

(3) Workforce Security

(a) Identify the extent of authorization each class of workforce members will require when accessing electronic protected health information, considering the criticality and sensitivity of the information to be handled.

        (b) Workforce member, contractors and others shall access only those areas and the applicable health information to which they are authorized.

        (c) Ensure appropriate training is completed before access to MIS components is granted or reinstated.

    (4) Information Systems Activity Review

        (a) Assign personnel to conduct a regular review of electronic protected health information systems' activities.

        (b) Reviewers should have appropriate technical skills to access and interpret audit logs correctly.

    (5) Contingency Plan

        (a) Identify the hardware, software, applications and information sets that receive, manipulate, store and/or transmit electronic protected health information. Define information sets for the purpose of criticality rating.

        (b) Identify backup methods and materials to be used, and the frequency of performing backups

        (c) Monitor storage and removal of backups and ensure all applicable access controls are enforced.

4. Applicability and Scope. All health care facilities (clinics, satellite clinics, and sickbays) shall comply with the MIS operating guidelines as set forth. The MIS program described here contains the essential elements required at all CG facilities with medical personnel assigned and assigns responsibilities for the program's initiatives. The SHSO shall ensure all healthcare providers and support staff; which include Medical Officers, Dental Officers, Pharmacy Officers, Health Services Administrators, HSs; HSDs and Medical and Dental contractors; shall participate. Information technology is not static in nature but rapidly changing and dynamic, and requires the diligence of all concerned to create and maintain a sound program.

5. Objectives.

    a. The Director of Health and Safety Commandant (CG-11) has established a MIS that provides necessary tools and capabilities to assist in making sound business decisions for those Commands having healthcare facilities.

    b. Identify and justify resources required to maintain a quality MIS.

c. Establish access and connectivity for CG-wide comprehensive utilization of AHLTA, ensuring local DoD host site affiliation for electronic referrals and consultations and access to the Central Data Repository for all military health system beneficiary medical records.

d. Establish and maintain clinic and sickbay Microcomputer Allowance Lists (MAL) that provide appropriate access to medical information systems for managing clinical and administrative operations.

e. Establish a standardized equipment list for peripherals. (e.g. pharmacy printers, Lab barcode readers, thin terminal clients devices, etc.).

f. Identify systems training requirements and ensure required education and training standards are established and maintained.

g. Provide direction as new adjuncts to existing programs are developed and deployed.

h. Participate in DoD sponsored software and product development for use in the medical arena.

6. Definitions.

a. The short list of acronyms and definitions below is provided for clarification of Chapter 14 terms:

(1) Intranet. A privately owned network based on the Transmission Control Protocol/Internet Protocol (TCP/IP) suite.

(2) Internet. A voluntary interconnected global network of computers based upon the TCP/IP protocol suite, originally developed by the U.S. Department of Defense Advanced Research Projects Agency.

(3) NIPERNET. Non-Classified Internet Protocol Routing Network. The Defense Information Systems network (DISN) Internet line for unclassified DoD and federal agency Internet traffic.

(4) CGDN+. CG Data Network Plus. The secure CG-wide area network (WAN).

(5) Firewall. Security measure which blocks unwanted/unauthorized entry to computer systems from outside the internal system.

(6) Host (site). Medical facility where a CHCS server platform resides.

(7) TelNet. Telecommunications Network. A protocol that facilitates remote logins to host site server and functions via the Internet. Restricted by CG IT authorities.

(8) <u>IP address</u>. Internet Provider address. An assignable 32 bit numeric identifier, which designates a device's location on an intranet network or on the Internet.

(9) <u>LIU</u>. Local Area Network Interface Unit. Device designed to provide external access and interface with the local area network (LAN).

7. <u>Organizational Responsibilities</u>. A detailed list of Organizational responsibilities and actions for each will be published in the Medical Information Implementation Guide (MIIG).

B. Medical Information System.

1. Background. Information technology is dynamic in nature and rapidly changing. Commandant (CG-112) is responsible for ensuring that the Health, Safety, and Work-Life Directorate's MIS continues to evolve. The MIS has evolved from manual data collection systems to automated systems such as CLAMS to the DoD's hospital-based Composite Health Care System (CHCS). The advent of TRICARE in the mid 1990's necessitated integration of the CG's health care information with that of DoD's infrastructure.

2. Systems. The following outlines current automated information systems, applications and program components that come under the CG MIS program.

   a. Provider Graphic User Interface (PGUI) and AHLTA. A graphical user interface is software that makes CHCS easier to understand and use. The PGUI currently used in the CG will transition to AHLTA as DOD resolves the connectivity, efficiency, security, and other issues.

   b. Medical Readiness Reporting System (MRRS). Section C of this Chapter provides further details.

   c. Dental Common Access System (DENCAS). The Dental Common Access System is an enterprise-wide, world class e-business system that functions seamlessly between ship and shore to provide a complete picture of Navy and CG personnel dental readiness. DENCAS also provides an accurate, real-time, comprehensive administrative reporting system.

   d. Protected Health Information Management Tool (PHIMT).

      (1) The Privacy Rule of the Health Information Portability and Accountability Act (HIPAA) requires a covered entity (i.e., the CG Health Care Program) to maintain a history of when and to whom disclosures of Protected Health Information (PHI) are made for purposes other than for treatment, payment and health care operations. The covered entity must be able to provide an accounting of these disclosures to an individual upon their request. Authorizations and Restrictions to disclosures from an individual to a covered entity are included in the information that is required for accounting purposes. Disclosures that are permitted but also must be accounted for are those made within six years of the date of request, in the following 12 categories:

         (a) As required by law, statute, regulation or court orders.

         (b) For public health reports, communicable disease control, FDA reports, and OSHA reports.

         (c) To government authorities regarding victims of abuse or domestic violence.

(d) To health oversight agencies.

(e) To judicial or administrative proceedings through an order from a court or administrative tribunal (or a subpoena if notice to the individual is provided).

(f) As required by law or court order, to identify a suspect, or to alert law enforcement of a crime.

(g) To funeral directors, coroners or medical examiners as authorized by law.

(h) To facilitate organ, eye or tissue donation.

(i) For research, as approved by a Review Board.

(j) To prevent a serious threat to health or safety.

(k) For execution of the military mission and other essential government functions.

(l) To comply with workers' compensation laws.

(2) To comply with the requirements for accounting for disclosures, the TMA has developed and provided and electronic disclosure tracking tool. The Protected Health Information Management Tool (PHIMT) stores information about disclosures, Authorizations and Restrictions that are made for a particular patient. The PHIMT also has a functionality that can provide an accounting of disclosures by individual patient, upon request.

(3) Use of the PHIMT is password protected, and several user roles are defined:

(a) A regular user can create disclosures and Authorization/Restriction requests.

(b) A user administrator can add/modify users within their Service.

(c) A Privacy/Security Officer can approve/deny disclosures, Authorizations and Restrictions, and generate the associated letters.

(4) A User Guide and an Administrator Guide for the PHIMT can be accessed through the HIPAA Learning Management Tool at www.HIPAAtraining.tricare.osd.mil using the student ID and password used for the HIPAA Privacy training module.

C. <u>Medical Readiness Reporting System (MRRS).</u>

1. <u>Description.</u> The Medical Readiness Reporting System (MRRS) is the CG's medical readiness reporting system adopted from the Navy. It is designed for use by clinics, independent duty health services technicians and CG Personnel Service Center. MRRS contains the following functional elements:

    a. Immunization data.

    b. Primary Physical Exam data.

    c. Periodic Health Assessment data.

    d. Medical Readiness data.

    e. Blood type/ tests data.

    f. Visual Acuity/ insert requirements.

    g. Dental Exam and classification.

    h. Pre/Post Deployment History.

    i. **OMSEP Examination History**

    j. Forms.

    k. Health record tracking.

2. <u>Recorded tests.</u> MRRS is designed to track medical readiness parameters (e.g. HIV test, TST, DNA specimen submission, G6PD, sickle test, blood type, primary physical exam currency, periodic health assessment currency, **OMSEP examination currency** and immunizations). The system is tailored to meet all Department of Defense (DoD) and CG medical readiness reporting requirements.

3. <u>Questions related to MRRS.</u> Questions on policy related to MRRS may be directed to Commandant (CG-1121).

4. <u>Access Instructions.</u> Members requiring access to MRRS need to request permissions from their local (clinic) MRRS Security Officer. Upon completion of mandatory MRRS training, members will receive access to MRRS after faxing or sending via electronic mail a completed System Access Request, Form DD-2875 to the appropriate Security Officer. This form is available on the MRRS website at https://mrrs.sscno.nmci.navy.mil.

D. <u>Medical Information Implementation Guide (MIIG)</u>.

1. <u>Background</u>. The MIIG is a series of guides designed to assist commands in meeting the requirements of the Health Services MIS Program requirements and to augment policy that is outlined in the Medical Manual. Serving as both policy and guidelines, the MIIG utilizes the same principal used in the QI program (as contained in Chapter 13), by outlining administrative requirements and by providing direction and policy for addressing critical MIS issues. The exercises provide generic frameworks adaptable to local conditions. In some cases, clinics may be required to submit evidence of completing an exercise to the HSWL SC for data evaluation purposes.

2. <u>Responsibilities</u>.

   a. <u>Commandant (CG-112)</u>. Commandant (CG-112) develops exercises as needed on critical MIS issues for inclusion in the MIIG and posts them on http://www.uscg.mil/hq/cg1/cg112/cg1123/default.asp.

   b. <u>HSWL SC</u>. The HSWL SC ensures guides are available to Commands for all clinic personnel to complete and also reviews clinic's use of the MIIGs as part of the Operational Health Readiness Program.

   c. <u>Unit Health Services Administrators (HSA) & System Administrators (SA)</u>. Unit HSA & SA shall ensure all clinic staff promptly comply with all MIIG guides and maintain a complete, updated MIIG folder.

COAST GUARD MEDICAL MANUAL

COMDTINST M6000.1F CH-2 JUNE 2018

This Commandant Change Notice publishes revisions to the Coast Guard Medical Manual, COMDTINST M6000.1F. This Notice is applicable to all active duty and reserve Coast Guard members and the other Services Members assigned to duty with the Coast Guard.

This book is over 700 pages so we split it into two (2) Volumes. This is Volume 2. It contains Chapters 8 thru Chapter 14.

Why buy a book you can download for free? We print this so you don't have to.

We at 4th Watch Publishing Co. are former government employees, so we know how government employees actually use the standards. When a new standard is released, an engineer prints it out, punches holes and puts it in a 3-ring binder. While this is not a big deal for a 5 or 10-page document, many documents are over 100 pages and printing and binding a large document is a time-consuming effort. First you have to find a good clean (legible) copy and make sure it's the latest version (not always easy). Some documents on the web are missing pages or the image quality is so poor, they are difficult to read. We look over each document carefully and replace poor quality images by going back to the original source document. We proof each document to make sure it's all there – including all changes. If you find a good copy, you could print it using a network printer you share with 100 other people (typically its either out of paper or toner). If it's just a 10-page document, no problem, but if it's 250-pages, you will need to punch 3 holes in all those pages and put it in a 3-ring binder. Takes at least an hour.

4th Watch Publishing Co. prints these documents so engineers can focus on what they were hired to do – engineering. This is important because there are not as many engineers working in government as there used to be, so wasted time on clerical duties is unproductive. It's much more cost-effective to just order the latest version through Amazon.com.

4th Watch Publishing Co. is a Service Disabled Veteran Owned Small Business (SDVOSB). Check out our other titles at:

USGOVPUB.COM

List of Other Coast Guard Publications available on Amazon in 2019:

COMDTPUB P3120.l7B   Coast Guard Incident Management Handbook
COMDTINST M5810.1G   Military Justice Manual
CIM 10470 10G   Rescue and Survival Systems Manual
CIM M3010.11E   Emergency Management Manual, Vol 1. Emergency Management Planning
CIM 5000 7A, 7B   Shipboard Regulations Manual Part 1 & 2
CIM 3710 1H   Air Operations Manual
CIM 3710 4D   Helicopter Rescue Swimmer Manual
CIM 3010 24   Contingency Preparedness Planning Manual Volume 4
CIM 16500 21A   Aids to Navigation Manual - Seamanship
CIM 16500 25A   Aids to Navigation Manual - Structures
CIM 16500 3A   Aids to Navigation Manual – Technical
CIM 16500 2   Hydrographic Manual Fourth Edition
CIM 16114 32D   Boat Operations and Training (BOAT) Manual Volume 1
CIM 16114 33C   Boat Operations and Training (BOAT) Manual Volume 2
CIM 16114 28   Non-Standard Boat Operator's Handbook
CIM 16000 6   Marine Safety Manual, Vol. 1, Administration
CIM 16000 7B   Marine Safety Manual, Vol. 2: Materiel Inspection
CIM 16000 10A   Marine Safety Manual, Vol. 5: Investigations
CIM 16000 11   Marine Safety Manual, Vol. 6: Ports and Waterways Activities
CIM 11012 9   Shore Facilities Volume 1
CIM 13020 1G   Aeronautical Engineering Maintenance Management
CIM 13020 3A   Contractor's Flight and Ground Operations
CIM 13482 2B   Multiservice Helicopter Sling Load: Basic Operations and Equipment
CIM 13482 3A   Multiservice Helicopter Sling Load: Single-Point Load Rigging Procedures
CIM 13482 4A   Multiservice Helicopter Sling Load: Dual-Point Load
CIM 5000 3B   United States Coast Guard Regulations

Other related publications:

Sea Level Rise Maps U.S. East Coast 2100
Sea Level Rise Maps Gulf Coast 2040 – 2100
FEMA   Coastal Construction Manual Volume 1
FEMA   Coastal Construction Manual Volume 2
FEMA   Local Officials Guide for Coastal Construction
FEMA   Home Builder's Guide to Coastal Construction
Uniform Code of Military Justice (UCMJ)
DOJ   Justice Manual
DOJ   Electronic Crime Scene Investigation
DOJ   Prosecuting Computer Crimes
JAGMAN   Manual of the Judge Advocate General (NAVY)
MCM   Manual for Courts-Martial
DA PAM 27-9   Military Judges' Benchbook
NLSC 5800.01G   Naval Legal Service Command Manual
The Supremes   Rules of the Supreme Court of the United States